Instant Pot Soup, Stew, Chili & Curry Recipes

Super Healthy Chicken Soup

Makes: 4 servings
Preparation Time: 15 minutes
Cooking Time: 12 minutes

Ingredients:

- 2 tablespoons olive oil
- 3 celery stalks, chopped
- 3 large carrots, peeled and chopped
- 1 small yellow onion, chopped
- ¼ teaspoon dried oregano, crushed
- ¼ teaspoon dried thyme, crushed
- Salt and freshly ground black pepper, to taste
- 4 cups homemade chicken broth
- 1 cup water
- 1 lb. grass-fed cooked chicken, shredded
- 2 cups fresh kale, trimmed and chopped

Directions:

1. Place the oil in the Instant Pot and select "Sauté". Then add the celery, carrot and onion and cook for about 5 minutes.
2. Add herbs and black pepper and cook for about 1 minute.
3. Select the "Cancel" and stir in the broth and water.
4. Secure the lid and select "Soup" and just use the default time of 4 minutes.
5. Select the "Cancel" and carefully do a Quick release.

6. Remove the lid and stir in the chicken and kale. Select "Sauté" and cook for about
7. 1-2 minutes more.
8. Serve immediately.

Nutritional Information per Serving:

Calories: 318
Fat: 11.9g
Saturated Fat: 2.4g
Sodium: 938mg
Carbohydrates: 11.9g
Dietary Fiber: 2.5g
Sugar: 4.3g
Protein: 39.5g

Comforting Chicken Soup

Makes: 8 servings
Preparation Time: 20 minutes
Cooking Time: 25 minutes

Ingredients:

- 2½ pounds grass-fed boneless, skinless chicken thighs
- 1 (10-ounce) can sugar-free diced tomatoes and green chilies
- 1 (14½-ounce) can sugar-free diced tomatoes
- 10-ounce frozen mix veggies (yellow onion, celery, bell pepper)
- 8 cups homemade chicken broth
- 2 teaspoons chili powder

- 1 teaspoon garlic powder
- Salt and freshly ground black pepper, to taste
- ½ cup fresh cilantro, chopped

Directions:

1. In the pot of Instant Pot, add all ingredients except cilantro.
2. Secure the lid and select "Soup" and just use the default time of 25 minutes.
3. Select the "Cancel" and carefully do a Natural release.
4. Remove the lid and with a slotted spoon, transfer chicken thighs into a bowl.
5. With 2 forks, shred chicken thighs and then return to the pot.
6. Stir in cilantro and serve immediately.

Nutritional Information per Serving:

Calories: 354
Fat: 12.3g
Saturated Fat: 3.3g
Sodium: 1012mg
Carbohydrates: 11.3g
Dietary Fiber: 2.4g
Sugar: 0.7.5g
Protein: 47.6g

Fabulous Turkey Soup

Makes: 6 servings
Preparation Time: 15 minutes
Cooking Time: 30 minutes

Ingredients:

- 1 tablespoon olive oil
- 1 lb. lean ground turkey
- 1 small yellow onion, chopped
- 2 cups carrots, peeled and shredded
- ½ head cabbage, chopped
- 4 cups homemade chicken broth
- ¼ cup low-sodium soy sauce
- 1 teaspoon ground ginger
- Freshly ground black pepper, to taste

Directions

1. Place the oil in the Instant Pot and select "Sauté". Then add the turkey and cook for about 5 minutes or until browned completely.
2. Select "Cancel" and stir in the remaining ingredients.
3. Secure the lid and cook under "Manual" and "High Pressure" for about 25 minutes.
4. Select the "Cancel" and carefully do a Quick release.
5. Remove the lid and serve immediately.

Nutritional Information per Serving:

Calories: 193
Fat: 8.7g
Saturated Fat: 2.3g
Sodium: 1189mg
Carbohydrates: 9.7g
Dietary Fiber: 2.7g
Sugar: 5.3g
Protein: 20g

Mexican Inspired Beef Soup

Makes: 8 servings
Preparation Time: 15 minutes
Cooking Time: 15 minutes

Ingredients:

- 1 teaspoon olive oil
- 2 pounds grass-fed lean ground beef
- 1 (20-ounce)can sugar-free diced tomatoes with green chilies
- 8 ouncescream cheese
- ½ cupheavy cream
- 4 cups homemade beef broth
- 4garlic cloves,minced
- 2tablespoonschili powder
- 2teaspoonsground cumin
- Salt and freshly ground black pepper, to taste
- ½ cup cheddar cheese,shredded

Directions:

1. Place the oil in the Instant Pot and select "Sauté". Then add the beef and cook for about 8-10 minutes. Drain excess grease from pot.
2. Select "Cancel" and stir in the remaining ingredients except cheddar cheese.
3. Secure the lid and select "Soup" and just use the default time of 5 minutes.
4. Select the "Cancel" and carefully do a Natural release.
5. Serve hot with the topping of cheddar cheese.

Nutritional Information per Serving:

Calories: 416
Fat: 23.8g
Saturated Fat: 12.5g
Sodium: 834mg
Carbohydrates: 6.7g
Dietary Fiber: 1.9g
Sugar: 3.5g
Protein: 42.5g

Full-Meal Beef Soup

Makes: 6 servings
Preparation Time: 15 minutes
Cooking Time: 38 minutes

Ingredients:

- 1 tablespoon olive oil
- 1 lb. grass-fed lean ground beef
- 1 small yellow onion, chopped
- 1 tablespoon garlic, minced
- 2 teaspoons dried thyme, crushed
- 1 teaspoon ground cumin
- 3 cups fresh tomatoes, chopped finely
- ¾ pound fresh green beans, trimmed and cut into 1-inch pieces
- 4¼ cups homemade beef broth
- Salt and freshly ground black pepper, to taste
- ¼ cup parmesan cheese, grated freshly

Directions:

1. Place the oil in the Instant Pot and select "Sauté". Then add the beef and cook for about 5 minutes or until browned completely.
2. Add onion, garlic, thyme, cumin and cook for about 3 minutes.
3. Select the "Cancel" and stir in the tomatoes, green beans and broth.
4. Secure the lid and cook under "Manual" and "Low Pressure" for about 30 minutes.
5. Select the "Cancel" and carefully do a Quick release.
6. Remove the lid and stir in the salt and black pepper.
7. Serve immediately with the garnishing of the parmesan cheese.

Nutritional Information per Serving:

Calories: 303
Fat: 15.7g
Saturated Fat: 6.3g
Sodium: 960mg
Carbohydrates: 10.1g
Dietary Fiber: 3.5g
Sugar: 4.2g
Protein: 28.9g

Omega-3 Rich Salmon Soup

Makes: 8 servings
Preparation Time: 20 minutes
Cooking Time: 17 minutes

Ingredients:

- 2 pounds salmon fillets
- 2 tablespoons coconut oil

- 2 cups carrots, peeled and chopped
- 1 cup celery stalk, chopped
- 1 cup yellow onion, chopped
- 2 cups cauliflower, chopped
- 4 cups homemade chicken broth
- 1½ cups half-and-half
- Salt and freshly ground black pepper, to taste
- ¼ cup fresh parsley, chopped

Directions:

1. Arrange the trivet in the bottom of Instant Pot. Add 1 cup of water in Instant Pot.
2. Place the salmon fillets on top of trivet in a single layer.
3. Secure the lid and cook under "Manual" and "High Pressure" for about 8-9 minutes.
4. Select the "Cancel" and carefully do a Quick release.
5. Remove the lid and transfer the salmon onto a plate.
6. Cut the salmon into bite sized pieces.
7. Remove water and trivet from Instant Pot.
8. Place the coconut oil in the Instant Pot and select "Sauté". Then add the carrots, celery and onion and cook for about 5 minutes or until browned completely.
9. Select the "Cancel" and stir in the cauliflower and broth.
10. Secure the lid and cook under "Manual" and "High Pressure" for about 8 minutes.
11. Select the "Cancel" and carefully do a Natural release.
12. Remove the lid and stir in salmon pieces, half-and-half, salt and black pepper until well combined.
13. Serve immediately with the garnishing of parsley.

Nutritional Information per Serving:

Calories: 284
Fat: 16.4g
Saturated Fat: 7.4g
Sodium: 508mg
Carbohydrates: 8.3g
Dietary Fiber: 1.9g
Sugar: 3.2g
Protein: 26.8g

Hearty Bacon & Veggie Soup

Makes: 6 servings
Preparation Time: 15 minutes
Cooking Time: 23 minutes

Ingredients:

- 1 tablespoon olive oil
- 1 small yellow onion, chopped
- 2 garlic cloves, minced
- 1 head cauliflower, chopped roughly
- 1 green bell pepper, seeded and chopped
- Freshly ground black pepper, to taste
- 4 cups homemade chicken broth
- 2 cups cheddar cheese, shredded
- 1 cup half-and-half
- 6 cooked turkey bacon slices, chopped
- 4 dashes hot pepper sauce

Directions:

1. Place the oil in the Instant Pot and select "Sauté". Then add the onion and garlic and cook for about 3 minutes.
2. Select the "Cancel" and stir in cauliflower, bell pepper, salt, black pepper and broth.
3. Secure the lid and select "Soup" and just use the default time of 15 minutes.
4. Select the "Cancel" and carefully do a Quick release.
5. Remove the lid and stir in remaining ingredients.
6. Select "Sauté" and cook for about 5 minutes.
7. Serve immediately.

Nutritional Information per Serving:

Calories: 430
Fat: 32.6g
Saturated Fat: 15.4g
Sodium: 1444mg
Carbohydrates: 8.5g
Dietary Fiber: 1.7g
Sugar: 3.3g
Protein: 25.8g

Richly Cheesy Broccoli Soup

Makes: 6 servings
Preparation Time: 15 minutes
Cooking Time: 13 minutes

Ingredients:

- 2 tablespoons butter

- 2 medium carrots, peeled and chopped
- 1 small yellow onion, chopped
- 2 tablespoons almond flour
- 1 garlic clove, minced
- 3 cups homemade vegetable broth
- 5 cups broccoli florets
- 1 teaspoon dill weed
- 1 teaspoon smoked paprika
- Salt and freshly ground black pepper, to taste
- 4 American cheese slices, cut into pieces
- 1 cup colby jack cheese, shredded
- 1 cup pepper jack cheese, shredded
- ½ cup parmesan cheese, shredded
- 1 cup half-and-half

Directions:

1. Place the butter in the Instant Pot and select "Sauté". Then add the carrot and onion and cook for about 2-3 minutes.
2. Stir in flour and garlic and cook for about 1 minute, stirring continuously.
3. Stir in broth and cook for about 1 minute or until smooth, stirring continuously.
4. Select the "Cancel" and stir in the broccoli.
5. Secure the lid and cook under "Manual" and "High Pressure" for about 8 minutes.
6. Select the "Cancel" and carefully do a Quick release.
7. Remove the lid and immediately stir in dill weed, paprika, salt and black pepper.
8. Add cheeses and half-and-half and stir until melted and well combined.
9. Serve immediately.

Nutritional Information per Serving:

Calories: 354
Fat: 24.9g

Saturated Fat: 14g
Sodium: 1018mg
Carbohydrates: 13.1g
Dietary Fiber: 3g
Sugar: 4.2g
Protein: 17.8g

Aromatic Carrot Soup

Makes: 6 servings
Preparation Time: 15 minutes
Cooking Time: 12 minutes

Ingredients:

- 2tablespoonsolive oil
- 1small yellow onion,chopped
- 1garlic clove,minced
- ¼ teaspoon dried parsley, crushed
- ¼ teaspoon dried basil, crushed
- 1lb. carrots,peeled and chopped
- Salt and freshly ground black pepper, to taste
- 1(13½-ounce)can unsweetened coconut milk
- 3cupshomemade chicken broth
- 1tablespoonSriracha
- 3 tablespoons fresh cilantro, chopped

Directions:

1. Place the oil in the Instant Pot and select "Sauté". Then add the onion and garlic and cook for about 3 minutes.
2. Add garlic and cook for about 1 minute.
3. Add carrots, salt and black pepper and cook for about 2 minutes.
4. Select the "Cancel" and stir in coconut milk, broth and Sriracha sauce.
5. Secure the lid and cook under "Manual" and "High Pressure" for about 6 minutes.
6. Select the "Cancel" and carefully do a Natural release for about 10 minutes and then do a Quick release.
7. Remove the lid and with an immerse blender, puree the soup.
8. Serve immediately with the garnishing of cilantro.

Nutritional Information per Serving:

Calories: 245
Fat: 20.6g
Saturated Fat: 14.4g
Sodium: 489mg
Carbohydrates: 13.2g
Dietary Fiber: 3.5g
Sugar: 6.7g
Protein: 4.7g

Enticing Veggie Soup

Makes: 6 servings
Preparation Time: 20 minutes
Cooking Time: 13 minutes

Ingredients:

- 2 teaspoons olive oil

- 1 small yellow onion, chopped
- 1 tablespoon garlic, minced
- 1 teaspoon dried thyme, crushed
- 1 lb. fresh Baby Bella mushrooms, chopped
- 4 cups cauliflower, chopped
- 6 cups homemade vegetable broth
- ¾ cup parmesan cheese, grated

Directions:

1. Place the oil in the Instant Pot and select "Sauté". Then add the onion and garlic and cook for about 2-3 minutes.
2. Add mushrooms and cook for about 4-5 minutes.
3. Select the "Cancel" and stir in cauliflower and broth.
4. Secure the lid and cook under "Manual" and "High Pressure" for about 5 minutes.
5. Select the "Cancel" and carefully do a Natural release.
6. Remove the lid and with an immerse blender, puree the soup.
7. Select the "Sauté" and stir in parmesan cheese.
8. Cook for about 5 minutes.
9. Serve immediately.

Nutritional Information per Serving:

Calories: 151
Fat: 6.8g
Saturated Fat: 3g
Sodium: 1042mg
Carbohydrates: 10.4g
Dietary Fiber: 3.2g
Sugar: 4.2g
Protein: 13.4g

Gourmet Chicken Stew

Makes: 8 servings
Preparation Time: 15 minutes
Cooking Time: 31 minutes

Ingredients:

- 3 tablespoons Worcestershire sauce
- 2 tablespoons fresh lime juice
- 2 tablespoons paprika
- 1 teaspoon ground cumin
- 1 teaspoon ground turmeric
- Salt and freshly ground black pepper, to taste
- 4 grass-fed whole chicken legs (drumsticks and thighs separated into 8 pieces)
- 1 tablespoon coconut oil
- 1 cup yellow onion, sliced
- 3 garlic cloves, minced
- 2 tablespoons homemade tomato puree
- 2 cups homemade chicken broth
- ½ cup fresh parsley, chopped

Directions:

1. In a large bowl, add Worcestershire sauce, lime juice and spices.
2. Add chicken and generously coat with marinade.
3. Refrigerate to marinate for about 1 hour.
4. Remove chicken from bowl, reserving marinade.
5. Place the coconut oil in the Instant Pot and select "Sauté". Then add the chicken pieces in 2 batches and cook for about 2 minutes per side.
6. With a slotted spoon, transfer chicken into a bowl.

7. In the pot, add onion and garlic and cook for about 2-3 minutes.
8. Select the "Cancel" and stir in cooked chicken, reserved marinade, tomato puree and broth.
9. Secure the lid and cook under "Manual" and "High Pressure" for about 20 minutes.
10. Select the "Cancel" and carefully do a Natural release.
11. Remove the lid and stir in cilantro.
12. Serve immediately.

Nutritional Information per Serving:

Calories: 263
Fat: 10.8g
Saturated Fat: 3.9g
Sodium: 375mg
Carbohydrates: 5g
Dietary Fiber: 1.3g
Sugar: 2.3g
Protein: 34.8g

Earthy Chicken Stew

Makes: 6 servings
Preparation Time: 15 minutes
Cooking Time: 16 minutes

Ingredients:

- 1 tablespoon olive oil
- 1 lb. fresh cremini mushrooms, stemmed and quartered

- 1 small yellow onion, chopped
- 1 tablespoon sugar-free tomato paste
- 3 garlic cloves, minced
- 6 (5-ounce) grass-fed skinless, boneless chicken thighs
- 1 cup green olives, pitted and halved
- 2 cups fresh cherry tomatoes, halved
- 1 cup homemade chicken broth
- Salt and freshly ground black pepper, to taste
- ¼ cup fresh parsley, chopped

Directions:

1. Place the oil in the Instant Pot and select "Sauté". Then add the mushrooms and onion and cook for about 4-5 minutes.
2. Add tomato paste and garlic and cook for about 1 minute.
3. Select "Cancel" and stir in the chicken, olives, tomatoes and broth
4. Secure the lid and cook under "Manual" and "High Pressure" for about 9-10 minutes.
5. Select the "Cancel" and carefully do a Natural release.
6. Remove the lid and stir in salt, black pepper and parsley.
7. Serve immediately.

Nutritional Information per Serving:

Calories: 271
Fat: 10.3g
Saturated Fat: 2.6g
Sodium: 413mg
Carbohydrates: 9.3g
Dietary Fiber: 2.4g
Sugar: 3.9g
Protein: 35.5g

Classic Beef Stew

Makes: 8 servings
Preparation Time: 20 minutes
Cooking Time: 45 minutes

Ingredients:

- 2½ pounds grass-fed beef stew meat, cubed
- 3 zucchinis, chopped
- 1 pound small broccoli florets
- 2 garlic cloves, minced
- ¾ cup homemade chicken broth
- 2 tablespoons curry powder
- Salt and freshly ground black pepper, to taste
- 14 ounces unsweetened coconut milk
- ¼ cup fresh cilantro, chopped

Directions:

1. In the pot of Instant Pot, place all ingredients except coconut milk and cilantro and stir to combine.
2. Secure the lid and cook under "Manual" and "High Pressure" for about 45 minutes.
3. Select the "Cancel" and carefully do a Natural release for about 10 minutes and then do a Quick release.
4. Remove the lid and stir in coconut milk.
5. Serve immediately with the garnishing of cilantro.

Nutritional Information per Serving:

Calories: 419
Fat: 21.3g
Saturated Fat: 13.9g
Sodium: 219mg
Carbohydrates: 10.3g
Dietary Fiber: 3.9g
Sugar: 4g
Protein: 47.3g

Irresistible Lamb Stew

Makes: 6 servings
Preparation Time: 20 minutes
Cooking Time: 25 minutes

Ingredients:

- 1 tablespoon olive oil
- 1 small yellow onion, chopped
- 1 celery stalk, chopped
- 1 tablespoon garlic, minced
- 2 pound grass-fed lamb shoulder, trimmed and cubed into 2-inch size
- 2 cups fresh tomatoes, chopped finely
- 2 tablespoons sugar-free tomato paste
- 2-3 tablespoons fresh lemon juice
- 1 teaspoon dried oregano, crushed
- 1 teaspoon dried basil, crushed
- 2 leaves
- Salt and freshly ground black pepper, to taste

- ½ cup homemade chicken broth
- 1 large green bell pepper, seeded and cut into 8 slices
- 1 large red bell pepper, seeded and cut into 8 slices
- ¼ cup fresh parsley, minced

Directions:

1. Place the oil in the Instant Pot and select "Sauté". Then add the onion and garlic and cook for about 2 minutes.
2. Select "Cancel" and stir in the remaining ingredients except bell peppers and parsley.
3. Secure the lid and cook under "Manual" and "High Pressure" for about 15 minutes.
4. Select the "Cancel" and carefully do a Natural release for about 10 minutes and then do a Quick release.
5. Remove the lid and select "Sauté".
6. Stir in bell peppers and cook for about 6-8 minutes.
7. Serve immediately with the garnishing of parsley.

Nutritional Information per Serving:

Calories: 342
Fat: 3.9g
Saturated Fat: 4.4g
Sodium: 220mg
Carbohydrates: 8.5g
Dietary Fiber: 2g
Sugar: 5g
Protein: 44.4g

Veggie Lover's Stew

Makes: 10 servings
Preparation Time: 25 minutes
Cooking Time: 23 minutes

Ingredients:

- 2 tablespoons olive oil
- 1smallyellow onion, chopped finely
- 2celery stalks, chopped finely
- 3garlic cloves, minced
- 2 jalapeño peppers, chopped
- 1teaspoondriedsage, crushed
- 1teaspoondriedrosemary, crushed
- 2 teaspoons ground cumin
- 1½ pound fresh mushrooms, chopped
- 2large carrots, peeled and chopped
- 3cupsfresh green beans, trimmed and chopped
- 1 (15-ounce) can sugar-free diced tomatoes
- 2 ounces sugar-free tomato sauce
- 3cupshomemade vegetable broth
- 2 tablespoons fresh lemon juice
- Salt and freshly ground black pepper, to taste
- 2 tablespoons arrowroot starch
- 3 tablespoons water

Directions:

1. Place the oil in the Instant Pot and select "Sauté". Then add the onion and celery and cook for about 2 minutes.
2. Add garlic, jalapeño peppers, dried herbs and cumin and cook for about 1 minute.

3. Add mushrooms and cook for about 4-5 minutes.
4. Select "Cancel" and stir in the remaining ingredients except arrowroot starch and water.
5. Secure the lid and cook under "Manual" and "High Pressure" for about 15 minutes.
6. Select the "Cancel" and carefully do a Quick release.
7. Meanwhile, in a small bowl, dissolve arrowroot starch in water.
8. Remove the lid and stir in arrowroot starch mixture until well combined.
9. Serve hot.

Nutritional Information per Serving:

Calories: 94
Fat: 3.8g
Saturated Fat: 0.6g
Sodium: 372mg
Carbohydrates: 12g
Dietary Fiber: 3.5g
Sugar: 4.8g
Protein: 5.8g

Chili & Curry Recipes

Delightful Chicken Chili

Makes: 8 servings
Preparation Time: 25 minutes
Cooking Time: 19 minutes

Ingredients:

- 2 tablespoons olive oil
- 3 pounds grass-fed bone-in skin-on chicken thighs and drumsticks
- ¾ pound tomatillos, husks removed and quartered
- 2 Anaheim peppers, seeded and chopped roughly
- 2 Poblano peppers, seeded and chopped roughly
- 2 Serrano peppers, seeded and chopped roughly
- 1 medium yellow onion, chopped roughly
- 6 garlic cloves, peeled
- 1½ tablespoons ground cumin
- 1 tablespoon dried thyme
- Salt, to taste
- ½ cup fresh cilantro, chopped
- ½ cup homemade chicken broth
- 1 tablespoon fish sauce
- 2 tablespoon fresh lime juice
- 1/3 cup plain Greek yogurt

Directions:

1. Place the oil in the Instant Pot and select "Sauté". Then add chicken, tomatillos, peppers, garlic, cumin, thyme and salt and cook for about 3-4 minutes.
2. Select "Cancel" and stir in broth.
3. Secure the lid and cook under "Manual" and "High Pressure" for about 15 minutes.
4. Select the "Cancel" and carefully do a Natural release.
5. Remove the lid and with tongs, transfer chicken pieces into a bowl.
6. In the pot, add cilantro, fish sauce and lime juice and with a hand blender, blend the mixture until pureed.
7. Remove skin and bones from chicken pieces and shred the meat.
8. Return chicken into pot and stir to combine.
9. Serve immediately with the topping of yogurt.

Nutritional Information per Serving:

Calories: 403
Fat: 17g
Saturated Fat: 4g
Sodium: 404mg
Carbohydrates: 7.3g
Dietary Fiber: 1.6g
Sugar: 2.4g
Protein: 53.8g

Popular Turkey Chili

Makes: 8 servings
Preparation Time: 15 minutes
Cooking Time: 50 minutes

Ingredients:

- 1 tablespoon olive oil
- ½ largeyellow onion, chopped
- 8garlic cloves, minced
- 2½ pounds leanground turkey
- 1½ (15-ounce) canssugar-free diced tomatoeswith liquid
- 2 ounces sugar-free tomato paste
- 1(4-ounce) can green chilies with liquid
- 2 tablespoons Worcestershire sauce
- ¼ cup red chili powder
- 2 tablespoons ground cumin
- 1 tablespoon dried oregano, crushed
- Salt and freshly ground black pepper, to taste
- 1 large avocado, peeled, pitted and sliced

Directions:

1. Place the oil in the Instant Pot and select "Sauté". Then add the onion and celery and cook for about 5 minutes.
2. Add garlic and cook for about 1 minute.
3. Add turkey and cook for about 8-9 minutes.
4. Select "Cancel" and stir in remaining ingredients except avocado.
5. Secure the lid and select "Meat/Stew" and just use the default time of 35 minutes.
6. Select the "Cancel" and carefully do a Natural release.

7. Remove the lid and serve hot with the topping of avocado slices.

Nutritional Information per Serving:

Calories: 321
Fat: 18g
Saturated Fat: 4.6g
Sodium: 239mg
Carbohydrates: 12.3g
Dietary Fiber: 4.9g
Sugar: 4.2g
Protein: 30.4g

Budget Friendly Beef Chili

Makes: 6 servings
Preparation Time: 15 minutes
Cooking Time: 27 minutes

Ingredients:

- 1 tablespoon avocado oil
- ½ yellow onion, chopped
- 1 small red bell pepper, seeded and chopped
- Salt, to taste
- 4 garlic cloves, minced
- 2 tablespoons sugar-free tomato paste
- 2 pounds grass-fed lean ground beef
- 3 tablespoons chili powder

- 1 tablespoon ground cumin
- 1 tablespoon dried oregano, crushed
- 1 (14½-ounce) can sugar-free diced tomatoes, drained
- ½ cup homemade chicken broth
- 2 tablespoons fresh lemon juice.
- 1/3 cup cheddar cheese, shredded

Directions:

1. Place the oil in the Instant Pot and select "Sauté". Then add the onion, bell pepper and a pinch of salt and cook for about 3 minutes.
2. Stir in garlic and tomato paste and cook for about 1 minute.
3. Add beef and salt and cook for about 5-7 minutes.
4. Add spices and thyme and cook for about 1 minute.
5. Select "Cancel" and stir in tomatoes and broth.
6. Secure the lid and cook under "Manual" and "High Pressure" for about 15 minutes.
7. Select the "Cancel" and carefully do a Natural release.
8. Remove the lid and stir in lemon juice.
9. Serve hot with the topping of cheddar cheese.

Nutritional Information per Serving:

Calories: 360
Fat: 13.1g
Saturated Fat: 5.2g
Sodium: 280mg
Carbohydrates: 9.8g
Dietary Fiber: 3.3g
Sugar: 4.3g
Protein: 49.8g

Luxurious 2-Meat Chili

Makes: 8 servings
Preparation Time: 15 minutes
Cooking Time: 40 minutes

Ingredients:

- 1 tablespoon olive oil
- 1 lb. grass-fed ground beef
- 1 lb. ground pork
- 3 medium tomatillos, chopped
- ½ of small yellow onion, chopped
- 2 jalapeño peppers, chopped
- 2 garlic cloves, minced
- 1 (6-ounce) can sugar-free tomato sauce
- 1 tablespoon chili powder
- 1 tablespoon ground cumin
- Salt and freshly ground black pepper, to taste
- ¼ cup water
- ½ cup cheddar cheese, shredded

Directions:

1. Place the oil in the Instant Pot and select "Sauté". Then add the beef and pork and cook for about 5 minutes.
2. Remove extra grease from pot.
3. Select "Cancel" and stir in remaining ingredients except cheese.
4. Secure the lid and cook under "Manual" and "High Pressure" for about 35 minutes.
5. Select the "Cancel" and carefully do a Natural release.

6. Remove the lid and serve hot with the topping of cheddar cheese.

Nutritional Information per Serving:

Calories: 244
Fat: 12.2g
Saturated Fat: 4.7g
Sodium: 348mg
Carbohydrates: 3.7g
Dietary Fiber: 1.2g
Sugar: 1.4g
Protein: 28.9g

Awesome Bacon Chili

Makes: 4 servings
Preparation Time: 15 minutes
Cooking Time: 45 minutes

Ingredients:

- 4 bacon slices, chopped
- 1 red bell pepper, seeded and chopped
- ½ of small yellow onion, chopped
- 2 garlic cloves, minced
- 1 pound grass-fed ground beef
- 1½ tablespoons chili powder
- 1 tablespoon smoked paprika
- 2 teaspoons ground cumin

- Freshly ground black pepper, to taste
- 1 (14-ounce) can sugar-free fire roasted tomatoes
- 2 ounces sugar-free tomato sauce
- ¼ cup sour cream

Directions:

1. Place the bacon in the Instant Pot and select "Sauté". Cook for about 4 to 5 minutes or until crisp.
2. With a slotted spoon, transfer bacon onto a paper towel lined plate, leaving 2 tablespoons of grease in pot.
3. Add bell peppers, onion and garlic and cook for about 5 minutes.
4. Add beef and spices and cook for about 5 minutes.
5. Select "Cancel" and stir in cooked bacon, tomatoes and tomato sauce.
6. Secure the lid and select "Bean/Chili" and just use the default time of 30 minutes.
7. Select the "Cancel" and carefully do a Natural release.
8. Remove the lid and serve hot with the topping of sour cream.

Nutritional Information per Serving:

Calories: 447
Fat: 23g
Saturated Fat: 8.6g
Sodium: 840mg
Carbohydrates: 12.2g
Dietary Fiber: 3.8g
Sugar: 5.5g
Protein: 47.6g

Authentic Chicken Curry

Makes: 10 servings
Preparation Time: 20 minutes
Cooking Time: 23 minutes

Ingredients:

For Spice Paste:

- ¼ of small yellow onion, chopped roughly
- 4 small, dried red chilies
- ¾ cup unsweetened coconut, grated
- 1 teaspoon fennel seeds
- 1 teaspoon coriander seeds
- 1 teaspoon cumin seeds
- 1 teaspoon black pepper corns
- 1 teaspoon ground cinnamon
- 1 teaspoon ground turmeric
- ¼ cup water

For Chicken:

- 1 tablespoon coconut oil
- 1 small yellow onion, chopped
- 2 garlic cloves, minced
- 3 large tomatoes, chopped
- 3 pounds grass-fed skinless, boneless chicken thighs, cubed
- 1 tablespoon fresh lemon juice
- Pinch of salt
- ½ cup fresh parsley, chopped

Directions:

1. For spice paste, add the small onion and dried chilies in Instant Pot. Select "Sauté "and cook for about 2 minutes.
2. Transfer the onion mixture into a food processor.
3. In the pot, add coconut and spices and cook for about 1 minute.
4. Select "Cancel" and transfer the spice mixture into the food processor with onion mixture.
5. Add water and pulse until a smooth paste forms.
6. Place the oil in the Instant Pot and select "Sauté". Then add the onion and cook for about 4-5 minutes.
7. Add the garlic and spice paste and cook for about 2 minutes.
8. Add tomatoes and cook for about 2-3 minutes.
9. Select "Cancel" and stir in the remaining ingredients except parsley.
10. Secure the lid and cook under "Manual" and "High Pressure" for about 10 minutes.
11. Select the "Cancel" and carefully do a Natural release.
12. Remove the lid and stir in parsley.
13. Serve hot.

Nutritional Information per Serving:

Calories: 224
Fat: 8.5g
Saturated Fat: 4.8g
Sodium: 72mg
Carbohydrates: 5.3g
Dietary Fiber: 2g
Sugar: 2.5g
Protein: 31.6g

Bright Green Chicken Curry

Makes: 10 servings
Preparation Time: 15 minutes
Cooking Time: 22 minutes

Ingredients:

- 3 pounds grass-fed boneless, skinless chicken thighs, cut into 2-inch long, thin slices
- Salt, to taste
- 1 tablespoon olive oil
- 1 small yellow onion, sliced thinly
- 3 garlic cloves, crushed
- 1 cup coconut cream
- 4 tablespoons green curry paste
- 8 ounces unsweetened coconut milk
- 1 cup homemade chicken broth
- 1 tablespoon fish sauce
- 1 tablespoon soy sauce
- 12 ounces green beans, trimmed and cut into 2-inch pieces
- 1 tablespoon fresh lime juice
- ¼ cup fresh cilantro, chopped

Directions:

1. Season the chicken thighs with salt and set aside.
2. Place the oil in the Instant Pot and select "Sauté". Then add onion and garlic and cook for about 3 minutes.
3. Stir in coconut cream and curry paste and cook for about 5 minutes, stirring occasionally.
4. Select "Cancel" and stir in the chicken, coconut milk, broth and both sauces.

5. Secure the lid and cook under "Manual" and "High Pressure" for about 10 minutes.
6. Select the "Cancel" and carefully do a Quick release.
7. Remove the lid and select "Sauté".
8. Stir in the green beans and lime juice and cook for about 4 minutes.
9. Serve hot with the garnishing of cilantro.

Nutritional Information per Serving:

Calories: 369
Fat: 19.1g
Saturated Fat: 8.5g
Sodium: 685mg
Carbohydrates: 7g
Dietary Fiber: 1.9g
Sugar: 1.8g
Protein: 41.4g

Rustic Beef Curry

Makes: 10 servings
Preparation Time: 20 minutes
Cooking Time: 46 minutes

Ingredients:

- 3 pounds grass-fed beef brisket, cubed into 1 1 2-inch size
- Salt, to taste
- 1 tablespoon coconut oil

- 2 tablespoons curry paste
- 1 pound cauliflower florets
- 2 large carrots, peeled and chopped
- 1 small yellow onion, chopped
- 1½ cups unsweetened coconut milk
- 2 tablespoons fresh lime juice
- 2 tablespoons coconut aminoes
- 2 tablespoons fish sauce
- ½ cup fresh cilantro, chopped

Directions:

1. Season the beef cubes with salt and keep aside.
2. Place the oil in the Instant Pot and select "Sauté". Then add curry paste and cook for about 1 minute.
3. Add beef and cook for about 4 -5 minutes.
4. Select "Cancel" and stir in remaining ingredients except cilantro.
5. Secure the lid and select "Meat" and just use the default time of 35 minutes.
6. Select the "Cancel" and carefully do a Natural release.
7. Remove the lid and serve hot with the topping of sour cream.
8. Select the "Cancel" and carefully do a Natural release for about 10 minutes and then do a Quick release.
9. Remove the lid and serve hot with the garnishing of cilantro.

Nutritional Information per Serving:

Calories: 392
Fat: 20.2g
Saturated Fat: 12g
Sodium: 416mg
Carbohydrates: 8.1g
Dietary Fiber: 2.4g
Sugar: 3.4g
Protein: 43.6g

Stunning Lamb Curry

Makes: 4 servings
Preparation Time: 15 minutes
Cooking Time: 35 minutes

Ingredients:

- 1 pound grass-fed lamb shoulder, cut into bite sized pieces
- 1 tablespoon curry powder, divided
- ¼ cup unsweetened coconut milk
- 2 tablespoons coconut cream
- 1 tablespoon coconut oil
- 1 medium yellow onion, chopped
- ½ cup homemade chicken broth
- 1 tablespoon fresh lemon juice
- Salt and freshly ground black pepper, to taste
- 2 tablespoons fresh basil, chopped

Directions:

1. In a large bowl, add lamb, ½ tablespoon of curry powder, coconut milk and coconut cream and stir to combine. Keep aside for at least 20 minutes.
2. After 20 minutes, remove lamb from bowl, reserving cream mixture.
3. Place the oil and butter in the Instant Pot and select "Sauté". Then add the onion and garlic and cook for about 3-4 minutes.
4. Add remaining curry powder and cook for about 1 minute.
5. Add lamb and stir fry for about 5 minutes.
6. Select the "Cancel" and stir in broth, lemon juice, salt and black pepper.
7. Secure the lid and cook under "Manual" and "High Pressure" for about 20 minutes.
8. Select the "Cancel" and carefully do a Quick release.
9. Remove the lid and select "Simmer".

10. Stir in reserved cream mixture and cook for about 4-5 minutes, stirring occasionally.
11. Serve immediately with the garnishing of basil.

Nutritional Information per Serving:

Calories: 323
Fat: 18.5g
Saturated Fat: 10.7g
Sodium: 288mg
Carbohydrates: 4.8g
Dietary Fiber: 1.5g
Sugar: 1.9g
Protein: 33.5g

Flavorsome Fish Curry

Makes: 4 servings
Preparation Time: 15 minutes
Cooking Time: 12 minutes

Ingredients:

- 1 tablespoon olive oil
- 2 curry leaves
- 1 small yellow onion, chopped
- 2 garlic cloves, minced
- 2 tablespoons curry powder
- 2 teaspoons ground cumin
- 2 teaspoons ground coriander

- 1 teaspoon red chili powder
- ½ teaspoon ground turmeric
- 2 cups unsweetened coconut milk
- 1½ pounds salmon fillets, cut into bite sized pieces
- 1¼ cups tomatoes, chopped
- 1 Serrano pepper, seeded and chopped
- 1 tablespoon fresh lemon juice

Directions:

1. Place the oil in the Instant Pot and select "Sauté". Then add the curry leaves and cook for about 30 seconds.
2. Add onions and garlic and cook for about 4-5 minutes.
3. Add spices and cook for about 1½ minute.
4. Select "Cancel" and stir in coconut milk, fish, tomatoes and Serrano pepper.
5. Secure the lid and cook under "Manual" and "Low Pressure" for about 5 minutes.
6. Select the "Cancel" and carefully do a Natural release.
7. Remove the lid and stir in the lemon juice.
8. Serve hot.

Nutritional Information per Serving:

Calories: 559
Fat: 43.2g
Saturated Fat: 27.5g
Sodium: 106mg
Carbohydrates: 12.2g
Dietary Fiber: 4.2g
Sugar: 6.5g
Protein: 36.9g

Instant Pot Poultry Recipes

Delectable Cornish Hens

Makes: 4 servings
Preparation Time: 20 minutes
Cooking Time: 23 minutes

Ingredients:

- 2 Cornish hens, washed and pat dried
- Salt and freshly ground black pepper, to taste
- 2 tablespoons coconut oil
- 1 small yellow onion, chopped
- 2 celery stalks, chopped
- 1 large carrot, peeled and chopped
- 4 garlic cloves, chopped
- 2 teaspoons Worcestershire sauce
- 1 cup water

Directions:

1. Season the hens with salt and black pepper generously.
2. Place the oil in the Instant Pot and select "Sauté". Then add hens, 1 at a time and cook for about 2 minutes per side.
3. Select "Cancel" and arrange both hens in the Instant Pot.
4. Top with remaining ingredients.
5. Secure the lid and cook under "Manual" and "Medium-High Pressure" for about 15 minutes.
6. Select the "Cancel" and carefully do a Natural release.
7. Remove the lid and transfer hens onto a platter for about 5 minutes before serving.

8. Serve alongside vegetables.

Nutritional Information per Serving:

Calories: 249
Fat: 11.7g
Saturated Fat: 7.1g
Sodium: 167mg
Carbohydrates: 5.2g
Dietary Fiber: 1g
Sugar: 2.3g
Protein: 29.7g

Fuss-Free Whole Chicken

Makes: 3-4 servings
Preparation Time: 15 minutes
Cooking Time: 31 minutes

Ingredients:

- 1 (2½-pound) grass-fed whole chicken, neck and giblet removed
- 1 tablespoon cayenne pepper
- Salt and freshly ground black pepper, to taste
- 2 tablespoon olive oil
- 1½ cups homemade chicken broth

Directions:

1. Season the chicken with cayenne pepper, salt and black pepper generously.

2. Place the oil in the Instant Pot and select "Sauté". Then add chicken and cook for about 5-6 minute or until browned.
3. Select the "Cancel" and transfer the chicken onto a plate.
4. Arrange the trivet in the bottom of Instant Pot. Add chicken broth in Instant Pot.
5. Arrange the chicken on top of trivet, breast side up.
6. Secure the lid and cook under "Manual" and "High Pressure" for about 25 minutes.
7. Select the "Cancel" and carefully do a Natural release.
8. Remove the lid and place chicken onto a cutting board for about 10 minutes before carving.
9. With a sharp knife, cut chicken into desires sized pieces and serve.

Nutritional Information per Serving:

Calories: 507
Fat: 16.3g
Saturated Fat: 3.6g
Sodium: 504mg
Carbohydrates: 1.1g
Dietary Fiber: 0.4g
Sugar: 0.4g
Protein: 84.1g

Deliciously Spicy Whole Chicken

Makes: 6 servings
Preparation Time: 15 minutes
Cooking Time: 42 minutes

Ingredients:

- 1 tablespoon fresh rosemary, minced
- ½ tablespoon ground cumin
- ½ tablespoon cayenne pepper
- ½ tablespoon red pepper flakes, crushed
- Salt and freshly ground black pepper, to taste
- 1 (4-pound) grass-fed whole chicken, neck and giblet removed
- 2 tablespoon olive oil

Directions:

1. In a bowl, mix together rosemary and spices. Rub the chicken with spice mixture generously.
2. Place the oil in the Instant Pot and select "Sauté". Then add the chicken and cook for about 6-7 minutes or until browned from all sides.
3. Select the "Cancel". Secure the lid and select "Poultry" and just use the default time of 20 minutes.
4. Select the "Cancel" and carefully do a Quick release.
5. Remove the lid and flip the side of chicken.
6. Secure the lid and cook under "Manual" and "High Pressure" for about 15 minutes.
7. Select the "Cancel" and carefully do a Quick release.
8. Remove the lid and place chicken onto a cutting board for about 10 minutes before carving.
9. With a sharp knife, cut chicken into desires sized pieces and serve.

Nutritional Information per Serving:

Calories: 502
Fat: 14.1g
Saturated Fat: 3.3g
Sodium: 219mg
Carbohydrates: 0.8g
Dietary Fiber: 0.4g

Sugar: 0.1g
Protein: 87.8g

Christmas Special Chicken

Makes: 6 servings
Preparation Time: 20 minutes
Cooking Time: 31 minutes

Ingredients:

- 2 tablespoon olive oil
- 1teaspoonpaprika
- ½ teaspoon red pepper flakes, crushed
- ½ teaspoongarlic powder
- Salt and freshly ground black pepper, to taste
- 1 (4-pound) grass-fed whole chicken, neck and giblet removed
- 1 small yellow onion, quartered
- 3garlic cloves,peeled
- 3 fresh thymesprigs
- ½ lemon
- 1 cup water

Directions:

1. In a small bowl, mix together oil and spices. Keep aside.
2. Stuff the cavity of chicken with onion, garlic, thyme and lemon.

3. Rub the oil mixture over the breast of chicken, under the skin and over the skin.
4. Select "Sauté".
5. Place chicken into the Instant Pot, breast side down.
6. Carefully, rub the oil mixture on the back side of the chicken.
7. Cook the chicken for about 2 to 3 minutes per side.
8. Select the "Cancel" and place water around the chicken.
9. Secure the lid and cook under "Manual" and "High Pressure" for about 25 minutes.
10. Select the "Cancel" and carefully do a Natural release.
11. Remove the lid and place chicken onto a cutting board for about 10 minutes before carving.
12. With a sharp knife, cut chicken into desires sized pieces and serve.

Nutritional Information per Serving:

Calories: 509
Fat: 14g
Saturated Fat: 3.3g
Sodium: 220mg
Carbohydrates: 2.8g
Dietary Fiber: 0.9g
Sugar: 0.7g
Protein: 88.1g

Simplest Chicken Breasts

Makes: 10 servings
Preparation Time: 10 minutes
Cooking Time: 10 minutes

Ingredients:

- 3 pounds grass-fed chicken breasts
- 1 cup homemade chicken broth
- Salt, to taste

Directions:

1. Add all ingredients except cilantro to Instant Pot.
2. Secure the lid and select "Poultry" and just use the default time of 10 minutes.
3. Select the "Cancel" and carefully do a Natural release for about 5 minutes and then do a Quick release.
4. Remove the lid and place chicken breasts onto a cutting board for about 5 minutes before slicing.
5. Cut each breast unto desired sized slices and serve.

Nutritional Information per Serving:

Calories: 262
Fat: 10.2g
Saturated Fat: 2.8g
Sodium: 209mg
Carbohydrates: 0.1g
Dietary Fiber: 0g
Sugar: 0.1g
Protein: 39.9g

Juicy Chicken Breast

Makes: 3 servings
Preparation Time: 15 minutes
Cooking Time: 13 minutes

Ingredients:

- 3(6-ounce) grass-fed boneless, skinless chicken breasts
- ½ teaspoon garlic powder
- Salt and freshly ground black pepper, to taste
- 1 tablespoon coconut oil
- ¼ teaspoondried oregano, crushed
- ¼ teaspoondried basil, crushed
- 1cupwater

Directions:

1. Generously season the chicken with garlic powder, salt and black pepper.
2. Place the coconut oil in the Instant Pot and select "Sauté". Then add chicken breasts and cook for about 3-4 minute per side.
3. Select the "Cancel" and transfer chicken breasts onto a plate.
4. Arrange the trivet in the bottom of Instant Pot. Add water in Instant Pot.
5. Arrange the chicken on top of trivet.
6. Secure the lid and cook under "Manual" and "High Pressure" for about 5 minutes.
7. Select the "Cancel" and carefully do a Quick release.
8. Remove the lid and place chicken onto a cutting board for about 5 minutes before serving.

Nutritional Information per Serving:

Calories: 364
Fat: 17.1g
Saturated Fat: 7.4g
Sodium: 199mg
Carbohydrates: 0.4g

Dietary Fiber: 0.1g
Sugar: 0.1g
Protein: 49.3g

Incredible Chicken Thighs

Makes: 4 servings
Preparation Time: 15 minutes
Cooking Time: 21 minutes

Ingredients:

- 1 tablespoon olive oil
- 2 garlic cloves, minced
- 4 (4-ounce) grass-fed skinless, boneless chicken thighs
- Salt and freshly ground black pepper, to taste
- ½ cup sugar-free tomato sauce
- ¼ cup low-sodium soy sauce
- 2 tablespoons Erythritol
- 2 tablespoons fresh lemon juice
- 1 tablespoons arrowroot starch
- 1 tablespoons water
- 2 tablespoons fresh basil, chopped

Directions:

1. Place the oil in the Instant Pot and select "Sauté". Then add the garlic and cook for about 1 minute.
2. Add chicken and sprinkle thighs with salt and black pepper and cook for about 5 minutes or until browned from all sides.

3. Select "Cancel" and stir in tomato sauce, soy sauce, Erythritol and lemon juice.
4. Secure the lid and cook under "Manual" and "High Pressure" for about 10 minutes.
5. Select the "Cancel" and carefully do a Quick release.
6. Meanwhile, in a small bowl, dissolve arrowroot starch in water.
7. Remove the lid and select "Sauté".
8. Add arrowroot starch mixture, stirring continuously. Cook for about 4-5 minutes, stirring continuously.
9. Select "Cancel" and serve hot with the garnishing of basil.

Nutritional Information per Serving:

Calories: 195
Fat: 2.1g
Saturated Fat: 2.1g
Sodium: 1083mg
Carbohydrates: 12.6g
Dietary Fiber: 0.6g
Sugar: 10g
Protein: 26.9g

Exotic Chicken Thighs

Makes: 8 servings
Preparation Time: 15 minutes
Cooking Time: 18 minutes

Ingredients:

- 1 tablespoon olive oil
- 2 pounds grass-fed boneless, skinless chicken thighs
- 1 teaspoon red pepper flakes, crushed
- Salt and freshly ground black pepper, to taste
- 1 yellow onion, minced
- ½ cup sugar-free BBQ sauce
- ½ cup water
- 2 tablespoons fresh lemon juice

Directions:

1. In a bowl, mix together BBQ sauce, water and lemon juice. Set aside.
2. Place the oil in the Instant Pot and select "Sauté". Then add the chicken thighs and cook for about 2 minutes per side.
3. Stir in paprika, salt, and black pepper and cook for about 1 minute.
4. Select "Cancel" and stir in BBQ sauce mixture.
5. Secure the lid and cook under "Manual" and "High Pressure" for about 15 minutes.
6. Select the "Cancel" and carefully do a Natural release.
7. Remove the lid and serve hot.

Nutritional Information per Serving:

Calories: 261
Fat: 10.3g
Saturated Fat: 2.6g
Sodium: 294mg
Carbohydrates: 7.2g
Dietary Fiber: 0.5g
Sugar: 4.8g
Protein: 33g

Distinctive Chicken Drumsticks

Makes: 8 servings
Preparation Time: 20 minutes
Cooking Time: 20 minutes

Ingredients:

- 1 tablespoon coconut oil
- 1 large yellow onion, peeled, cut into wedges
- Salt, to taste
- 8 (6-ounce) grass-fed skin on chicken drumsticks
- ¼ teaspoon red chili powder
- Freshly ground black pepper, to taste
- 2/3 cup canned sugar-free diced tomatoes
- 8 garlic cloves, peeled
- 2 tablespoons fresh thyme leaves, minced
- 1 teaspoon fresh lemon zest, grated finely
- 2 tablespoons fresh lemon juice

Directions:

1. Place the oil in the Instant Pot and select "Sauté". Then add the onion and a little of salt and cook for about 2-3 minutes, stirring occasionally.
2. Add the chicken drumsticks, salt, chili powder ad black pepper and cook for about 2 minutes.
3. Select "Cancel" and stir in tomatoes, garlic, thyme, lemon zest and lemon juice.
4. Secure the lid and select "Poultry" and just use the default time of 15 minutes.
5. Select the "Cancel" and carefully do a Natural release for about 5 minutes and then do a Quick release.

6. Remove the lid and serve chicken drumsticks with pan gravy.

Nutritional Information per Serving:

Calories: 320
Fat: 11.6g
Saturated Fat: 4.1g
Sodium: 159mg
Carbohydrates: 3.9g
Dietary Fiber: 1g
Sugar: 1.3g
Protein: 47.4g

Asian Style Chicken Drumsticks

Makes: 10 servings
Preparation Time: 20 minutes
Cooking Time: 15 minutes

Ingredients:

- 1 cup coconut milk
- 1 thick fresh lemongrass stalk, outer skins and rough bottom removed and trimmed
- 4 garlic cloves, crushed
- 2 tablespoons low-sodium soy sauce
- 2 tablespoons fish sauce
- 1 teaspoon five spice powder
- 10 grass-fed skinless chicken drumsticks
- Salt and freshly ground black pepper, to taste

- 1 teaspoon coconut oil
- 1 large yellow onion, sliced thinly
- ¼ cup fresh cilantro, chopped
- 2 tablespoons fresh lime juice

Directions:

1. In a blender, add coconut milk, lemongrass, garlic, soy sauce, fish sauce and five-spice powder and pulse until a smooth sauce is formed.
2. Season chicken drumsticks with salt and black pepper evenly.
3. Place the oil in the Instant Pot and select "Sauté". Then add the onion and cook for about 3 minutes.
4. Select "Cancel" and stir in chicken drumsticks and sauce.
5. Secure the lid and cook under "Manual" and "High Pressure" for about 15 minutes.
6. Select the "Cancel" and carefully do a Quick release.
7. Remove the lid and stir in cilantro and lime juice.
8. Serve hot.

Nutritional Information per Serving:

Calories: 147
Fat: 8.8g
Saturated Fat: 6.2g
Sodium: 511mg
Carbohydrates: 3.5g
Dietary Fiber: 0.9g
Sugar: 1.8g
Protein: 13.8g

Impressive Chicken Leg Quarters

Makes: 4 servings
Preparation Time: 15 minutes
Cooking Time: 20 minutes

Ingredients:

- 1 cup homemade chicken broth
- 4 (8-ounce) grass-fed skinless chicken leg quarters
- 1 teaspoon garlic powder
- Salt and freshly ground black pepper, to taste
- 2 tablespoons olive oil

Directions:

1. Arrange the trivet in the bottom of Instant Pot. Add broth in Instant Pot.
2. Season chicken leg quarters with garlic powder, salt and black pepper.
3. Place the chicken leg quarters on top of trivet in a single layer.
4. Secure the lid and cook under "Manual" and "High" for about 20 minutes.
5. Preheat the oven to broil.
6. Select the "Cancel" and carefully do a Quick release.
7. Remove the lid and with tongs, transfer the chicken leg quarters onto a parchment paper lined baking sheet.
8. Coat chicken leg quarters with oil evenly and broil for about 5 minutes per side.
9. Serve hot.

Nutritional Information per Serving:

Calories: 457
Fat: 33.7g
Saturated Fat: 8.2g
Sodium: 594mg
Carbohydrates: 0.8g
Dietary Fiber: 0.1g
Sugar: 0.3g
Protein: 39.8g

Restaurant Style Chicken Leg Quarters

Makes: 4 servings
Preparation Time: 20 minutes
Cooking Time: 27 minutes

Ingredients:

- 1 tablespoon olive oil
- 4 (8-ounce) grass-fed skinless chicken leg quarters
- 1 small yellow onion, chopped finely
- 2 teaspoons hot paprika
- ½ teaspoon red pepper flakes, crushed
- ½ cup homemade chicken broth
- 1 medium tomato, chopped
- Salt, to taste
- ½ cup sour cream

Directions:

1. Place the oil in the Instant Pot and select "Sauté". Then add the chicken leg quarters and cook for about 4--5 minutes.
2. With a slotted spoon, transfer the chicken leg quarters into a plate.
3. Select the "Cancel" and stir in onion, paprika, red pepper flakes.
4. Top with chicken leg quarters, followed by tomato and sprinkle with salt.
5. Secure the lid and cook under "Manual" and "High Pressure" for about 8 minutes.
6. Select the "Cancel" and carefully do a Natural release.
7. Remove the lid and with tongs, transfer the chicken leg quarters into a plate.
8. Select "Sauté" and cook for about 10 minutes.
9. In a bowl, add the sour cream and ¼ cup of hot liquid from Instant Pot and beat until smooth.
10. Add the sour cream mixture into Instant Pot and stir to combine.
11. Stir in cooked chicken and cook for about 3-4 minutes.
12. Select the "Cancel" and serve hot.

Nutritional Information per Serving:

Calories: 568
Fat: 31.5g
Saturated Fat: 12.2g
Sodium: 758mg
Carbohydrates: 6.8g
Dietary Fiber: 3.2g
Sugar: 1.8g
Protein: 64.7g

Super-Simple Chicken Wings

Makes: 4 servings
Preparation Time: 20 minutes
Cooking Time: 20 minutes

Ingredients:

- 1 1/3 pounds grass-fed chicken wings
- 4 tablespoon taco seasoning
- Salt, to taste

Directions:

1. In a shallow dish, mix together taco seasoning and salt.
2. Add chicken wings and coat with seasoning mixture evenly.
3. Arrange the trivet in the bottom of Instant Pot. Add 1 cup of water in Instant Pot.
4. Place the wings on top of trivet in a single layer.
5. Secure the lid and cook under "Manual" and "High Pressure" for about 10 minutes.
6. Preheat the oven to broil.
7. Select the "Cancel" and carefully do a Quick release.
8. Remove the lid and transfer chicken wings onto a parchment paper lined baking sheet and broil for about 5-10 minutes.
9. Serve hot.

Nutritional Information per Serving:

Calories: 295
Fat: 11.2g
Saturated Fat: 3.1g
Sodium: 330mg
Carbohydrates: 1.1g
Dietary Fiber: 0.3g

Sugar: 0.4g
Protein: 43.7g

Flavored Chicken Wings

Makes: 4 servings
Preparation Time: 20 minutes
Cooking Time: 23 minutes

Ingredients:

- 1½ pounds grass-fed chicken wings
- ¼ cup tomato puree
- 1 tablespoon Erythritol
- 1 tablespoon fresh lemon juice
- Salt and freshly ground black pepper, to taste

Directions:

1. Arrange the trivet in the bottom of Instant Pot. Add 1 cup of water in Instant Pot.
2. Place chicken wings on top of trivet, standing vertically.
3. Secure the lid and cook under "Manual" and "High Pressure" for about 10 minutes.
4. Preheat the oven to broil.
5. Select the "Cancel" and carefully do a Quick release.
6. Meanwhile in a bowl, add remaining ingredients and beat until well combined.

7. Remove the lid and transfer chicken wings into the bowl of sauce.
8. Coat the wings with sauce generously.
9. Arrange the chicken wings onto a parchment paper lined baking sheet and broil for about 5 minutes.
10. Serve hot with remaining sauce.

Nutritional Information per Serving:

Calories: 330
Fat: 12.7g
Saturated Fat: 3.5g
Sodium: 190mg
Carbohydrates: 5.3g
Dietary Fiber: 0.3g
Sugar: 4.6g
Protein: 49.5g

Traditional Moroccan Chicken

Makes: 8 servings
Preparation Time: 20 minutes
Cooking Time: 25 minutes

Ingredients:

- 1 teaspoon olive oil
- 3 pounds grass-fed bone-in chicken leg quarters
- 1 pound cherry tomatoes, crushed slightly

- 2 garlic cloves, crushed
- 1 teaspoon dried oregano, crushed
- ¼ teaspoon red pepper flakes, crushed
- Salt, to taste
- ½ cup homemade chicken broth
- ½ cup green olives, pitted
- 1 tablespoon fresh basil leaves, torn

Directions:

1. Place the oil in the Instant Pot and select "Sauté". Then add the chicken leg quarters and cook for about 4-5 minutes.
2. With a slotted spoon, transfer the chicken leg quarters into a plate.
3. In the Instant Pot, add crushed cherry tomatoes with all juice, garlic, oregano, red pepper flakes and salt and cook for about 1 minute, scraping up the brown bits from bottom.
4. Select the "Cancel" and stir in the cooked chicken and broth.
5. Secure the lid and cook under "Manual" and "High Pressure" for about 13-14 minutes.
6. Select the "Cancel" and carefully do a Quick release.
7. Remove the lid and select "Sauté".
8. Stir in olives and basil and cook for about 5 minutes.
9. Select the "Cancel" and serve hot.

Nutritional Information per Serving:

Calories: 424
Fat: 33.6g
Saturated Fat: 9.4g
Sodium: 288mg
Carbohydrates: 3.2g
Dietary Fiber: 1.1g
Sugar: 1.6g
Protein: 28.3g

Succulent Chicken Platter

Makes: 4 servings
Preparation Time: 20 minutes
Cooking Time: 23 minutes

Ingredients:

- 1 tablespoon olive oil
- 2 (4-ounce) grass-fed skinless, boneless chicken breasts
- Salt and freshly ground black pepper, to taste
- 1 small yellow onion, chopped
- 1 garlic clove, minced
- 1¼ cups homemade chicken broth
- 1½ tablespoons arrowroot starch
- 3½ tablespoons water, divided
- ½ cup cheddar cheese, shredded
- 2 ounces cream cheese, cubed
- 2 cups small broccoli florets

Directions:

1. Place the oil in the Instant Pot and select "Sauté". Then add the chicken breasts and cook for about 4-5 minutes.
2. With a slotted spoon, transfer the chicken breasts into a plate.
3. Add onion and cook for about 2-3 minutes.
4. Add garlic and cook for about 1 minute.
5. Select the "Cancel" and stir in the cooked chicken and broth.
6. Secure the lid and cook under "Manual" and "High Pressure" for about 5 minutes.
7. Select the "Cancel" and carefully do a Quick release.

8. Remove the lid and with tongs, transfer chicken breasts onto a cutting board.
9. With a sharp knife, cut chicken into desired sized pieces.
10. Meanwhile in a small bowl, dissolve arrowroot starch in 1½ tablespoons of water.
11. Now, select "Sauté" of Instant Pot.
12. Add arrowroot mixture, stirring continuously.
13. Add cheddar cheese and cream cheese and cook until melted completely, stirring continuously.
14. Meanwhile in a large microwave-safe bowl, add broccoli and 2 tablespoons of water and microwave on High for about 3-4 minutes.
15. Add chopped chicken and broccoli in Instant Pot and stir well.
16. Simmer for about 4-5 minutes.
17. Select the "Cancel" and serve hot.

Nutritional Information per Serving:

Calories: 253
Fat: 15.7g
Saturated Fat: 7.5g
Sodium: 443mg
Carbohydrates: 8.4g
Dietary Fiber: 1.7g
Sugar: 1.8g
Protein: 20.3g

Midweek Dinner Chicken

Makes: 4 servings
Preparation Time: 15 minutes
Cooking Time: 8 minutes

Ingredients:

- 1 tablespoon olive oil
- 1 small yellow onion, chopped
- 1 jalapeño pepper, seeded and chopped
- 1 cup cooked grass-fed chicken, chopped
- 1½ pound cabbage, sliced into thin strips
- ½ cup homemade chicken broth
- ½ tablespoon fresh lemon juice
- Salt and freshly ground black pepper, to taste

Directions:

1. Place the oil in the Instant Pot and select "Sauté". Then add the onion and cook for about 3 minutes.
2. Add chicken and cook for about 2 minutes.
3. Select the "Cancel" and add cabbage and broth to the chicken and stir.
4. Secure the lid and cook under "Manual" and "High Pressure" for about 3 minutes.
5. Select the "Cancel" and carefully do a Quick release.
6. Remove the lid and stir in lemon juice, salt and black pepper.
7. Serve hot.

Nutritional Information per Serving:

Calories: 139
Fat: 5g
Saturated Fat: 0.9g
Sodium: 188mg
Carbohydrates: 11.9g
Dietary Fiber: 4.8g
Sugar: 6.4g
Protein: 3.2g

Best-Ever Chicken Meatballs

Makes: 8 servings
Preparation Time: 20 minutes
Cooking Time: 30 minutes

Ingredients:

- 1½ pounds grass-fed ground chicken
- ¾ cup almond meal
- 2 scallions, sliced thinly
- 2 garlic cloves, minced
- Salt, to taste
- 5 tablespoons butter, divided
- 6 tablespoons hot sauce

Directions:

1. In a large bowl, add chicken, almond meal, scallions, garlic and salt and with your hands, mix until well combined.

2. With greased hands, make 24 equal sized balls from mixture.
3. Place 2 tablespoons of butter in the Instant Pot and select "Sauté". Then add the meatballs in batches and cook for about 4-5 minutes.
4. Meanwhile, for sauce: in a microwave-safe bowl, add remaining butter and hot sauce and microwave until butter is melted completely.
5. Select the "Cancel" and place all browned meatballs in the Instant Pot and top with sauce evenly.
6. Secure the lid and select "Poultry" and just use the default time of 15-20 minutes.
7. Select the "Cancel" and carefully do a Quick release.
8. Remove the lid and serve hot.

Nutritional Information per Serving:

Calories: 280
Fat: 18g
Saturated Fat: 6.7g
Sodium: 430mg
Carbohydrates: 2.6g
Dietary Fiber: 1.3g
Sugar: 0.6g
Protein: 26.7g

Thanksgiving Dinner Turkey

Makes: 8 servings
Preparation Time: 20 minutes
Cooking Time: 50 minutes

Ingredients:

- 2 tablespoons butter
- 1 (11-pound) whole turkey, necks and gibbets removed
- 3 fresh thyme sprigs
- 2 - 3 fresh rosemary sprigs
- 1 cup homemade chicken broth
- 2 tablespoons fresh lemon juice

Directions:

1. Season turkey with salt and black pepper evenly.
2. Place butter in a larger Instant Pot and select "Sauté". Then add the turkey and cook until browned.
3. Select the "Cancel" and transfer turkey onto a tray.
4. Stuff the cavity of turkey with herb sprigs and tie up the legs together.
5. In the pot of Instant Pot, place turkey and pour broth and lemon juice on top.
6. Secure the lid and cook under "Manual" and "High Pressure" for about 45 minutes.
7. Select the "Cancel" and carefully do a Natural release for about 10 minutes and then do a Quick release.
8. Remove the lid and place turkey onto a cutting board for about 15-20 minutes before carving.
9. Cut turkey into desired sized slices and serve.

Nutritional Information per Serving:

Calories: 1096
Fat: 34.4g
Saturated Fat: 12.2g
Sodium: 554mg
Carbohydrates: 1.2g
Dietary Fiber: 0.6g
Sugar: 0.2g
Protein: 183.4g

Moist Turkey Breast

Makes: 2 servings
Preparation Time: 20 minutes
Cooking Time: 14 minutes

Ingredients:

- 2 (8-ounce) turkey breast fillets
- 2 garlic cloves, minced
- 1tablespoonfresh sage, minced
- Salt and freshly ground black pepper, to taste

Directions:

1. Arrange the trivet in the bottom of Instant Pot. Add 1 cup of water in Instant Pot.
2. Place the turkey fillets on top of trivet in a single layer.
3. Secure the lid and select "Poultry" and just use the default time of 10 minutes.
4. Select the "Cancel" and carefully do a Quick release.
5. Remove the lid and serve.

Nutritional Information per Serving:

Calories: 337
Fat: 3.3g
Saturated Fat: 1.2g
Sodium: 78mg
Carbohydrates: 1.9g
Dietary Fiber: 2.3g
Sugar: 0.3g
Protein: 74.3g

Celebratory Turkey Breast

Makes: 8 servings
Preparation Time: 20 minutes
Cooking Time: 14 minutes

Ingredients:

- 1 cup homemade chicken broth
- 1 teaspoon dried rosemary, crushed
- 1 teaspoon dried parsley, crushed
- 1 teaspoon dried thyme, crushed
- 1 teaspoon dried sage, crushed
- 1 teaspoon red pepper flakes, crushed
- Salt and freshly ground black pepper, to taste
- 1 (6-7-pound) turkey breast

Directions:

1. Arrange the trivet in the bottom of Instant Pot. Add broth in Instant Pot.
2. In a bowl, mix together herbs, red pepper flakes, salt and black pepper.
3. Rub turkey breast with herb mixture generously.
4. Place the turkey breast on top of trivet.
5. Secure the lid and select "Poultry" and just use the default time of 45 minutes.
6. Select the "Cancel" and carefully do a Natural release.
7. Preheat the oven to broil.
8. Remove the lid and transfer turkey breast onto a baking sheet.
9. Broil for about 5-10 minutes or until desired doneness.
10. Remove from oven and place the turkey breast onto a cutting board for about 5-10 minutes.
11. Cut into desired sized slices and serve.

Nutritional Information per Serving:

Calories: 368
Fat: 4.7g
Saturated Fat: 0.1g
Sodium: 311mg
Carbohydrates: 0.4g
Dietary Fiber: 0.2g
Sugar: 0.1g
Protein: 85g

Holiday Dinner Turkey Quarters

Makes: 4 servings
Preparation Time: 20 minutes
Cooking Time: 43 minutes

Ingredients:

- 2 (2½-pound) turkey quarters
- Salt and freshly ground black pepper, to taste
- 2 tablespoons olive oil, divided
- 1 medium onion, chopped
- 3 garlic cloves, minced
- 1 large carrot, peeled and chopped
- 1 celery stalk, chopped
- 2 bay leaves
- A pinch of dried rosemary
- A pinch of dried thyme

- A pinch of dried sage
- 1 tablespoon fresh lemon juice
- 1 cup homemade chicken broth
- 3 tablespoons arrowroot starch
- 2 tablespoons cold water

Directions:

1. Season the turkey quarters with salt and black pepper generously.
2. Place 1 tablespoon of oil in Instant Pot and select "Sauté". Then add the turkey quarters and cook for about 4-5 minutes per side.
3. Select the "Cancel" and transfer turkey quarters onto a plate.
4. Now, place remaining oil in Instant Pot and select "Sauté". Then add the onion and garlic and cook for about 1 minute.
5. Add carrot and celery and cook for about 5-7 minutes.
6. Add bay leaves, herbs, salt and black pepper and cook for about 1 minute.
7. Add lemon juice and scrape the brown bits.
8. Select the "Cancel" and stir in turkey quarters and broth.
9. Secure the lid and cook under "Manual" and "High Pressure" for about 20 minutes.
10. Select the "Cancel" and carefully do a Natural release for about 10 minutes and then do a Quick release.
11. Remove the lid and transfer the turkey quarters onto a platter.
12. In a small bowl, dissolve the arrowroot starch in water.
13. For gravy: select "Sauté" and slowly, add the arrowroot starch mixture, stirring continuously.
14. Cook for about 2-3 minutes or until desired thickness, stirring continuously.
15. Select the "Cancel" and transfer the gravy into a serving bowl.
16. Serve turkey quarters alongside the gravy.

Nutritional Information per Serving:

Calories: 910
Fat: 47.6g

Saturated Fat: 13.7g
Sodium: 489mg
Carbohydrates: 9.7g
Dietary Fiber: 1.2g
Sugar: 1.8g
Protein: 111.9g

Dinner Party Duck

Makes: 3 servings
Preparation Time: 20 minutes
Cooking Time: 43 minutes

Ingredients:

- 1 (3½-pounds) wild duck
- Salt and freshly ground black pepper, to taste
- 2 tablespoons butter
- 1 lemon, halved
- 2 sprigs fresh rosemary
- ½ cup homemade chicken broth

Directions:

1. With a fork, prick the skin of duck.
2. Season the body and cavity of duck with salt and black pepper evenly.
3. Stuff the cavity of duck with lemon halves and rosemary sprigs and tie up the legs together.

4. Place the butter in Instant Pot and select "Sauté". Then add the duck and cook for about 4 to 5 minutes or until browned from all sides.
5. Select the "Cancel" and remove grease from pot.
6. Add broth into Instant Pot.
7. Secure the lid and cook under "Manual" and "High Pressure" for about 25 minutes.
8. Select the "Cancel" and carefully do a Natural release.
9. Remove the lid and transfer the duck onto a cutting board.
10. Cut into desired sized pieces and serve.

Nutritional Information per Serving:

Calories: 858
Fat: 50.5g
Saturated Fat: 20.3g
Sodium: 434mg
Carbohydrates: 1.1g
Dietary Fiber: 0.5g
Sugar: 0.2g
Protein: 94g

Enjoyable Duck Legs

Makes: 4 servings
Preparation Time: 20 minutes
Cooking Time: 50 minutes

Ingredients:

- 4 (7-ounce) duck legs
- Salt and freshly ground black pepper, to taste

- ½ tablespoon olive oil
- ¼ cup carrot, peeled and chopped
- ¼ cup celery stalk, chopped
- ¼ cup yellow onion, chopped
- 3 garlic cloves, chopped
- 1 cup homemade chicken broth
- 2 tablespoons fresh lemon juice
- 1/8 teaspoon dried sage
- 1/8 teaspoon dried thyme
- 2 tablespoons fresh parsley, chopped

Directions:

1. Generously season the duck legs with salt and black pepper.
2. Place oil in Instant Pot and select "Sauté". Then add the turkey legs and cook for about 10 minutes.
3. Select the "Cancel" and transfer duck legs onto a plate.
4. Remove grease from pot, leaving about 1 teaspoon inside.
5. Select "Sauté" and cook carrot, celery, onion and garlic for about 1-2 minutes.
6. Select the "Cancel" and stir in duck legs, broth, dried herbs, salt and black pepper.
7. Secure the lid and cook under "Manual" and "High Pressure" for about 40-45 minutes.
8. Select the "Cancel" and carefully do a Quick release.
9. Remove the lid and with tongs, transfer turkey legs onto a platter.
10. With a stick blender, blend the onion mixture in the pot.
11. Select "Sauté" and cook for about 2-3 minutes.
12. Select the "Cancel" and transfer the gravy into a serving bowl.
13. Serve duck legs alongside gravy.

Nutritional Information per Serving:

Calories: 391
Fat: 14g
Saturated Fat: 3.1g
Sodium: 457mg
Carbohydrates: 2.8g
Dietary Fiber: 0.6g
Sugar: 1.1g
Protein: 59.4g

Stunning Quail Dinner

Makes: 4 servings
Preparation Time: 20 minutes
Cooking Time: 23 minutes

Ingredients:

- 2 (5-ounce) whole quails, cleaned and emptied and rinsed
- Salt and freshly ground black pepper, to taste
- 1 fresh thyme bunch
- 1 fresh rosemary bunch
- ½ cup homemade chicken broth
- 3½ ounces bacon, chopped
- ½ small yellow onion, chopped finely
- 1/8 teaspoon dried rosemary
- 1/8 teaspoon dried thyme
- 1 bay leaf

Directions:

1. Season the quails with salt and black pepper slightly.
2. Stuff the cavity of quails with fresh herbs bunches.
3. Place the oil in the Instant Pot and select "Sauté". Then add the bacon, onion, dried herbs, bay leaf, salt and black pepper and cook for about 2-3 minutes.
4. Place the quails in pot, breast-side down and cook for about 4-5 minutes or until browned completely.
5. Flip the side and now, place quails, breast-side up.
6. Select the "Cancel" and add the broth in pot.
7. Secure the lid and cook under "Manual" and "High Pressure" for about 7-9 minutes.
8. Select the "Cancel" and carefully do a Quick release.
9. Remove the lid and with tongs, transfer quails onto a plate. Then, remove the herb sprigs from cavity.
10. Strain the liquid into a bowl.
11. Return the broth in Instant pot and select "Sauté".
12. Cook for about 3-4 minutes.
13. Add the quail and cook for about 2 minutes, pouring the sauce over quails occasionally.
14. Remove the lid and serve the quails with sauce.

Nutritional Information per Serving:

Calories: 586
Fat: 31g
Saturated Fat: 6.9g
Sodium: 1415mg
Carbohydrates: 2.7g
Dietary Fiber: 0.4g
Sugar: 0.9g
Protein: 70.8g

Instant Pot Meat Recipes

Magically Tasty Chuck Roast

Makes: 6 servings
Preparation Time: 15 minutes
Cooking Time: 35 minutes

Ingredients:

For Rub:

- 2 tablespoons finely ground coffee
- 1 tablespoon cocoa powder
- 1 tablespoon smoked paprika
- 1 teaspoon ground ginger
- 1 teaspoon red chili powder
- 1 teaspoon red pepper flakes, crushed
- Salt and freshly ground black pepper, to taste
- 2 pound grass-fed beef chuck roast, trimmed and cut into 1½-inch cubes

For Sauce:

- 1 cup homemade beef broth
- ½ cup brewed coffee
- 1 medium yellow onion, chopped
- 2 tablespoons fresh lemon juice
- Salt and freshly ground black pepper, to taste

Directions:

1. For rub: in a small bowl, mix together all ingredients except roast.
2. Rub chuck roast with rub mixture generously.
3. For sauce: in a food processor, add all ingredients and pulse until smooth.
4. In the pot of Instant Pot, place roast and top with sauce evenly.
5. Secure the lid and select "Meat/Stew" and just use the default time of 35 minutes.
6. Select the "Cancel" and carefully do a Natural release.
7. Remove the lid and transfer the roast onto a platter.
8. With 2 forks, shred the meat.
9. Top with sauce and serve.

Nutritional Information per Serving:

Calories: 573
Fat: 42.8g
Saturated Fat: 17g
Sodium: 259mg
Carbohydrates: 3.7g
Dietary Fiber: 1.4g
Sugar: 1.2g
Protein: 41.1g

Family Dinner Chuck Roast

Makes: 8 servings
Preparation Time: 10 minutes
Cooking Time: 1 hour 25 minutes

Ingredients:

- 3 pound grass-fed beef chuck roast, trimmed and cut into large chunks
- 1 large yellow onion, sliced
- 6 garlic cloves
- 2 (4-ounce) cans of green chilies
- 1 tablespoon oregano
- Salt and freshly ground black pepper, to taste
- ¼ cup fresh lime juice
- ¾ cup water

Directions:

1. In the pot of Instant Pot, add all ingredients and stir to combine.
2. Secure the lid and cook under "Manual" and "High Pressure" for about 1 hour.
3. Select the "Cancel" and carefully do a Natural release.
4. Remove the lid and transfer the roast onto a plate.
5. With 2 forks, shred the meat and return into Instant Pot.
6. Now, select "Sauté" and cook for about 20-25 minutes or until desired doneness of sauce.
7. Select the "Cancel" and serve hot.

Nutritional Information per Serving:

Calories: 642
Fat: 47.4g
Saturated Fat: 18.9g
Sodium: 244mg
Carbohydrates: 5.1g
Dietary Fiber: 0.7g
Sugar: 1.8g
Protein: 44.9g

Irresistible Chuck Roast

Makes: 12 servings
Preparation Time: 10 minutes
Cooking Time: 1 hour 50 minutes

Ingredients:

- 6 pound grass-fed chuck roast
- 1 tablespoon garlic, minced
- 1 tablespoonWorcestershiresauce
- 2 teaspoons onion powder
- Salt and freshly ground black pepper, to taste
- 1½ cups homemade beef broth

Directions:

1. In the pot of Instant Pot, add all ingredients and stir to combine.
2. Secure the lid and cook under "Manual" and "High Pressure" for about 1½ hour.
3. Select the "Cancel" and carefully do a Natural release for about 15 minutes and then do a Quick release.
4. Remove the lid and through a meshstrainer, strain liquid into a bowl.
5. Transfer meat into a bowl and with 2 forks, shred it.
6. meat and return into Instant Pot.
7. Now, select "Sauté" and cook for about 15--20 minutes or until desired doneness of sauce.
8. Select the "Cancel" and serve hot.

Nutritional Information per Serving:

Calories: 498
Fat: 19g

Saturated Fat: 6.9g
Sodium: 271mg
Carbohydrates: 0.9g
Dietary Fiber: 0g
Sugar: 0.5g
Protein: 75.6g

Mexican Beef Brisket

Makes: 6 servings
Preparation Time: 20 minutes
Cooking Time: 40 minutes

Ingredients:

- 2½ pounds grass-fed beef boneless brisket, trimmed and cut into 1½-inch cubes
- 1 tablespoon chili powder
- Salt and freshly ground black pepper, to taste
- 1 tablespoon ghee
- 1 medium onion, sliced thinly
- 6 garlic cloves, peeled and smashed
- 1 tablespoon sugar-free tomato paste
- ½ cup roasted tomato salsa
- ½ cup homemade beef broth

Directions:

1. In a large bowl, add beef, chili powder, salt and black pepper and toss to coat well.
2. Place the ghee in the Instant Pot and select "Sauté". Then add the onions and cook for about 3-4 minutes.
3. Stir in the garlic and tomato paste and cook for about 1 minute.
4. Select the "Cancel" and stir in beef, salsa and broth.
5. Secure the lid and select "Meat/Stew" and just use the default time of 35 minutes.
6. Select the "Cancel" and carefully do a Natural release.
7. Remove the lid and serve hot.

Nutritional Information per Serving:

Calories: 402
Fat: 14.3g
Saturated Fat: 5.8g
Sodium: 345mg
Carbohydrates: 6g
Dietary Fiber: 1g
Sugar: 2g
Protein: 58.4g

Sunday Special Flank Steak

Makes: 4 servings
Preparation Time: 20 minutes
Cooking Time: 23 minutes

Ingredients:

- 1 pound grass-fed flank steaks, trimmed and cut into ¼-inch thick strips
- Salt and freshly ground black pepper, to taste
- ½ tablespoon olive oil
- 2 garlic cloves, minced
- ¼ cup water
- ¼ cup low-sodium soy sauce
- 2 tablespoons fresh lemon juice
- 1 tablespoon Erythritol
- 1 tablespoon arrowroot starch
- 1½ tablespoons cold water
- 2 tablespoons fresh parsley, chopped

Directions:

1. Season steak with salt and black pepper evenly.
2. Place the oil in the Instant Pot and select "Sauté". Then add the steak, salt and black pepper and cook for about 5 minutes.
3. Transfer the beef into a bowl.
4. In Instant Pot, add garlic and sauté for about 1 minute. A???
5. Select the "Cancel" and stir in beef, ¼ cup of water, soy sauce, lemon juice and Erythritol.
6. Secure the lid and cook under "Manual" and "High Pressure" for about 12 minutes.
7. Select the "Cancel" and carefully do a Quick release.
8. Meanwhile in a small bowl, dissolve arrowroot starch in cold water.
9. Remove the lid and select the "Sauté".
10. Add arrowroot mixture in Instant Pot, stirring continuously.
11. Cook for about 4-5 minutes or until desired thickness.
12. Stir in parsley and serve hot.

Nutritional Information per Serving:

Calories: 252
Fat: 11.3g

Saturated Fat: 4.2g
Sodium: 947mg
Carbohydrates: 7.3g
Dietary Fiber: 0.2g
Sugar: 5g
Protein: 32.8g

Mouth Watering Spare Ribs

Makes: 12 servings
Preparation Time: 15 minutes
Cooking Time: 19 minutes

Ingredients:

- 10 pounds grass-fed spare ribs, cut into serving pieces
- 2 teaspoons paprika
- Salt and freshly ground black pepper, to taste
- 3 teaspoons olive oil
- 2 small yellow onions, sliced
- 2 cups sugar-free ketchup
- 1 cup homemade beef broth
- 2 tablespoons fresh lemon juice
- 2 teaspoons Worcestershire sauce

Directions:

1. For sauce: in a bowl, add ketchup, broth, lemon juice and Worcestershire sauce and mix until well combined.

2. Generously season the ribs with paprika, salt and black pepper.
3. Place the oil in the Instant Pot and select "Sauté". Then add the ribs and cook for about 3-4 minutes or until browned completely.
4. Select the "Cancel" and place onion over ribs.
5. Top with sauce evenly.
6. Secure the lid and cook under "Manual" and "High Pressure" for about 15 minutes.
7. Select the "Cancel" and carefully do a Natural release.
8. Remove the lid and serve hot.

Nutritional Information per Serving:

Calories: 834
Fat: 35.5g
Saturated Fat: 13.2g
Sodium: 758mg
Carbohydrates: 11.7g
Dietary Fiber: 0.5g
Sugar: 9.9g
Protein: 110.5g

Ultimate Short Ribs

Makes: 8 servings
Preparation Time: 15 minutes
Cooking Time: 63 minutes

Ingredients:

- ½ cup almond flour
- Salt and freshly ground black pepper, to taste
- 3¼ pounds grass-fed beef short ribs

- 3 tablespoons unsalted butter, divided
- 1 small yellow onion, chopped
- 2 garlic cloves, minced
- 1 tablespoon fresh rosemary, chopped
- ½ cup homemade beef broth

Directions:

1. In a large bowl, mix together almond flour, salt and black pepper.
2. Generously add beef ribs and coat with flour mixture. Shake off excess mixture.
3. Place 1 tablespoon of butter in the Instant Pot and select "Sauté". Then add the ribs and cook for about 6-8 minutes or until browned completely.
4. Transfer the beef ribs into a bowl.
5. Add remaining butter and onion and cook for about 2-3 minutes.
6. Add garlic and rosemary and cook for about 1 minute.
7. Stir in broth and water and cook for about 1 minute.
8. Select "Cancel" and stir in the beef ribs.
9. Secure the lid and cook under "Manual" and "High Pressure" for about 50 minutes.
10. Select the "Cancel" and carefully do a Quick release.
11. Remove the lid and transfer ribs onto a serving platter.
12. Top with cooking liquid and serve.

Nutritional Information per Serving:

Calories: 466
Fat: 24.4g
Saturated Fat: 9.4g
Sodium: 212mg
Carbohydrates: 2.9g
Dietary Fiber: 1.1g
Sugar: 0.4g
Protein: 55.2g

Extremely Delicious Short Ribs

Makes: 4 servings
Preparation Time: 15 minutes
Cooking Time: 45 minutes

Ingredients:

- 2 pounds grass-fed beef short ribs, cut into 3-4-inch segments.
- Salt and freshly ground black pepper, to taste
- 1½ teaspoons olive oil
- 1 cup yellow onion, chopped
- 1 teaspoon garlic, minced
- ½ cup homemade beef broth
- 1/3 cup sugar-free ketchup
- 1½ tablespoons low-sodium soy sauce
- 1 tablespoon Worcestershire sauce
- 1 teaspoon Erythritol
- 1 fresh thyme sprig

Directions:

1. Season ribs with salt and pepper.
2. Place the oil in the Instant Pot and select "Sauté". Then add the ribs and cook for about 4 to 5 minutes or until browned completely.
3. Transfer the beef ribs into a bowl.
4. Add onions and cook for about 3-4 minutes.
5. Add garlic and cook for about 1 minute.
6. Select the "Cancel" and place ribs over onion.
7. For sauce: in a bowl, add remaining ingredients except thyme sprig and mix until well combined.
8. Pour sauce over ribs evenly and top with thyme sprig.

9. Secure the lid and select "Meat/Stew" and just use the default time of 35 minutes.
10. Select the "Cancel" and carefully do a Natural release for about 5 minutes and then do a Quick release.
11. Discard thyme sprig and serve hot.

Nutritional Information per Serving:

Calories: 422
Fat: 18g
Saturated Fat: 6.5g
Sodium: 1305mg
Carbohydrates: 9.2g
Dietary Fiber: 0.6g
Sugar: 7.4g
Protein: 54.6g

Classic French Beef Meal

Makes: 8 servings
Preparation Time: 20 minutes
Cooking Time: 1 hour 7 minutes

Ingredients:

For Beef:

- 3½ pound grass-fed beef chuck roast, trimmed and cubed into 2-inch size
- 3 garlic cloves, minced
- 1 tablespoon mixed dried herbs, crushed (of your choice)

- Salt and freshly ground white pepper, to taste
- 2 tablespoons unsalted butter
- 1 small yellow onion, chopped
- 2¼ cups homemade beef broth
- 2 tablespoons fresh lemon juice
- 4 large carrots, peeled and cut into 1-inch pieces

For Mushroom Gravy:

- 4 tablespoons unsalted butter
- 4 ounces cremini mushrooms, sliced
- ½ teaspoon dried thyme, crushed
- ¼ cup homemade beef broth
- 1 tablespoon fresh lemon juice
- ½ cup sour cream

Directions:

1. Put beef in a bowl. Add beef, garlic, mixed herbs, salt and white pepper and toss to coat well.
2. Place the butter in the Instant Pot and select "Sauté". Then add the onion and cook for about 4-5 minutes.
3. Add the broth and lemon juice and cook for about 1-2 minutes scraping the brown bits from the bottom.
4. Select the "Cancel" and place the beef over the onion, followed by broth.
5. Secure the lid and cook under "Manual" and "High Pressure" for about 40 minutes.
6. Select the "Cancel" and carefully do a Quick release.
7. Remove the lid and stir in the carrot.
8. Select "Sauté" and cook for about 10 minutes.
9. Transfer the beef mixture into a large bowl and cover with a piece of foil to keep warm.
10. For gravy: Place the butter in the Instant Pot and select "Sauté". Then add the mushrooms, thyme and wine and cook for about 10 minutes.
11. Select the "Cancel" and stir in the sour cream.

12. Immediately, place mushroom gravy over beef mixture and serve.

Nutritional Information per Serving:

Calories: 866
Fat: 67.4g
Saturated Fat: 29.5g
Sodium: 481mg
Carbohydrates: 6.7g
Dietary Fiber: 1.4g
Sugar: 2.8g
Protein: 54.9g

Favorite Thai Beef Dinner

Makes: 5 servings
Preparation Time: 20 minutes
Cooking Time: 32 minutes

Ingredients:

- 1 tablespoon olive oil
- 1 pound grass-fed beef chuck roast, trimmed and cut into thin strips
- Salt and freshly ground black pepper, to taste
- 1 small yellow onion, chopped
- 2 garlic cloves, minced
- Pinch of red pepper flakes, crushed
- ½ cup homemade beef broth
- ¼ cup low-sodium soy sauce
- 1 tablespoon Erythritol

- 1 tablespoon arrowroot starch
- 1½ tablespoons cold water
- ¾ pound broccoli florets
- 2 tablespoons water
- 2 tablespoons fresh cilantro, chopped

Directions:

1. Place the oil in the Instant Pot and select "Sauté". Then add the beef, salt and black pepper and cook for about 5 minutes.
2. Transfer the beef into a bowl.
3. Now, add onion and cook for about 4-5 minutes.
4. Add garlic and red pepper flakes and cook for about 1 minute.
5. Add broth, soy sauce and Erythritol and stir well.
6. Select the "Cancel" and stir in beef.
7. Secure the lid and cook under "Manual" and "High Pressure" for about 12 minutes.
8. Select the "Cancel" and carefully do a Quick release.
9. Meanwhile in a small bowl, dissolve arrowroot starch in cold water.
10. Remove the lid and select the "Sauté".
11. Add arrowroot mixture in Instant Pot, stirring continuously.
12. Cook for about 4-5 minutes or until desired thickness.
13. Meanwhile in a large microwave safe bowl, add broccoli and 2 tablespoons of water and microwave on High for about 3-4 minutes.
14. Add broccoli in Instant Pot and stir well.
15. Select the "Cancel" and serve with the garnishing of cilantro.

Nutritional Information per Serving:

Calories: 398
Fat: 28.4g
Saturated Fat: 10.5g
Sodium: 862mg
Carbohydrates: 11.6g

Dietary Fiber: 2.2g
Sugar: 5.6g
Protein: 27.2g

Colourful Beef & Peppers Combo

Makes: 5 servings
Preparation Time: 20 minutes
Cooking Time: 30 minutes

Ingredients:

- 1 tablespoon olive oil
- 1 pound grass-fed boneless beef, trimmed and sliced into thin strips
- Salt and freshly ground black pepper, to taste
- 2 cups tomatoes, chopped finely
- 1½ cups sugar-free tomato sauce
- 3 garlic cloves, minced
- 1 teaspoon dried rosemary, crushed
- 1 cup water
- 1 large green bell pepper, seeded and sliced into ½-inch thick strips
- 1 large red bell pepper, seeded and sliced into ½-inch thick strips
- 1 large yellow bell pepper, seeded and sliced into ½-inch thick strips

Directions:

1. Place the oil in the Instant Pot and select "Sauté". Then add the beef, a little salt and black pepper and cook for about 5 minutes.
2. Select the "Cancel" and transfer the beef into a bowl.
3. Now, add tomatoes, tomato sauce, garlic, rosemary, salt, black pepper and water in the bottom of pressure cooker and stir to combine.
4. Place beef on top, followed by bell peppers.
5. Secure the lid and cook under "Manual" and "High Pressure" for about 25 minutes.
6. Select the "Cancel" and carefully do a Quick release.
7. Remove the lid and serve hot.

Nutritional Information per Serving:

Calories: 249
Fat: 9g
Saturated Fat: 2.6g
Sodium: 452mg
Carbohydrates: 12.9g
Dietary Fiber: 3.1g
Sugar: 8.6g
Protein: 30g

Pure Comfort Ground Beef

Makes: 6 servings
Preparation Time: 15 minutes
Cooking Time: 43 minutes

Ingredients:

- 2 tablespoons coconut oil
- 2 medium carrots, peeled and chopped
- 2 celery sticks, chopped
- 1 small yellow onion, chopped finely
- Salt, to taste
- 2¼ pounds grass-fed ground beef
- 4 garlic cloves, chopped finely
- 2 tablespoons low-sodium soy sauce
- 1 teaspoon fish sauce
- 1 teaspoon paprika
- ½ teaspoon ground cinnamon
- 2 (14-ounce) cans sugar-free diced tomatoes with juice

Directions:

1. Place the oil in the Instant Pot and select "Sauté". Then add the carrot, celery and onion and cook for about 5 minutes.
2. Add the beef and cook for about 2-3 minutes.
3. Add garlic, both sauces and spices and cook for about 5 minutes.
4. Select the "Cancel" and stir in tomatoes with juice.
5. Secure the lid and cook under "Manual" and "High Pressure" for about 20 minutes.
6. Select the "Cancel" and carefully do a Natural release.
7. Remove the lid and select "Sauté".
8. Cook for about 5-10 minutes or until desired thickness of sauce.
9. Select the "Cancel" and serve hot.

Nutritional Information per Serving:

Calories: 299
Fat: 11.6g
Saturated Fat: 6g

Sodium: 401mg
Carbohydrates: 7.3g
Dietary Fiber: 2g
Sugar: 4.1g
Protein: 40.3g

Yummy Beef Meatballs

Makes: 6 servings
Preparation Time: 20 minutes
Cooking Time: 39 minutes

Ingredients:

- 1½ pounds grass-fed ground beef
- 2 teaspoons adobo seasoning
- Salt and freshly ground black pepper, to taste
- 1 tablespoon olive oil
- 4 small tomatoes, chopped roughly
- 10 mini bell peppers, seeded and halved
- 1 small yellow onion, chopped roughly
- 4 garlic cloves, peeled
- 1 cup sugar-free tomato sauce
- ½ teaspoon red pepper flakes, crushed

Directions:

1. In a bowl, add beef, adobo seasoning, salt and black pepper and mix well.
2. Make golf ball sized balls from mixture.

3. Place the oil in the Instant Pot and select "Sauté". Then add the meatballs and cook for about 3-4 minutes or until browned completely.
4. Select the "Cancel" and transfer meatballs into a bowl.
5. In the pot of Instant Pot, place remaining ingredients and top with meatballs.
6. Secure the lid and select "Meat/Stew" and just use the default time of 35 minutes.
7. Select the "Cancel" and carefully do a Natural release.
8. Remove the lid and with a slotted spoon, transfer the meatballs onto a plate.
9. With an immersion blender, blend the vegetable mixture until smooth.
10. Add meatballs, salt and black pepper into sauce and gently stir to combine.
11. Serve immediately.

Nutritional Information per Serving:

Calories: 223
Fat: 7.5g
Saturated Fat: 2.3g
Sodium: 726mg
Carbohydrates: 11.6g
Dietary Fiber: 2.5g
Sugar: 7.4g
Protein: 27.7g

Tempting Beef Meatloaf

Makes: 8 servings
Preparation Time: 20 minutes
Cooking Time: 23 minutes

Ingredients:

- 2 pounds grass-fed ground beef
- 1¼ cups fire roasted salsa, divided
- 1 large yellow onion, chopped
- 1 organic egg
- ¼ cup arrowroot starch
- 1 teaspoon ground cumin
- 1 teaspoon red chili powder
- 1 teaspoon paprika
- Salt and freshly ground black pepper, to taste
- 1 tablespoon avocado oil

Directions:

1. In a large bowl, add all ingredients except ¼ cup of salsa and oil and mix until well combined.
2. Shape the mixture into a loaf, pressing firmly.
3. Place the oil in the Instant Pot and select "Sauté". Then carefully, place the meatloaf and top with remaining salsa.
4. Secure the lid and select "Meat/Stew" and just use the default time of 35 minutes.
5. Select the "Cancel" and carefully do a Quick release.
6. Remove the lid and carefully, transfer the meatloaf onto serving platter.
7. Cut into desired sized slices and serve.

Nutritional Information per Serving:

Calories: 265
Fat: 8g
Saturated Fat: 2.9g
Sodium: 319mg

Carbohydrates: 9.6g
Dietary Fiber: 0.9g
Sugar: 2.2g
Protein: 35.5g

Potluck Favorite Meatloaf

Makes: 6 servings
Preparation Time: 15 minutes
Cooking Time: 23 minutes

Ingredients:

- 1 small yellow onion, chopped roughly
- 6-8 garlic cloves, chopped
- 2 teaspoons fresh rosemary
- 2 teaspoons fresh marjoram
- Salt and freshly ground black pepper, to taste
- 2 pounds grass-fed ground beef
- ¼ cup feta cheese, crumbled

Directions:

1. In a food processor, add onion and pulse until chopped well.
2. Place chopped onion in a paper towel and squeeze out all the liquid.
3. Return into food processor with garlic, herbs, salt and black pepper and pulse until garlic is minced.
4. Add ground beef and pulse until well combined.
5. Place mixture into a loaf pan evenly and press firmly.

6. With a piece of foil, cover the loaf pan tightly and with a fork, poke a few vent holes into foil.
7. Arrange the trivet in the bottom of Instant Pot. Add 1½ cups of water in Instant Pot.
8. Arrange the meatloaf on top of trivet.
9. Secure the lid and cook under "Manual" and "High Pressure" for about 20 minutes.
10. Select the "Cancel" and carefully do a Natural release.
11. Preheat the oven to broiler.
12. Remove loaf pan and place onto a wire rack to cool for about 15 minutes.
13. Carefully, remove meatloaf from pan and transfer onto a broiler pan.
14. Broil for about 2-3 minutes.
15. Remove from oven and immediately, top with feta cheese.
16. Cut into desired sized slices and serve.

Nutritional Information per Serving:

Calories: 232
Fat: 8.2g
Saturated Fat: 3.4g
Sodium: 148mg
Carbohydrates: 2.3g
Dietary Fiber: 0.4g
Sugar: 0.6g
Protein: 35.4g

Weekend Dinner Pork Shoulder

Makes: 6 servings
Preparation Time: 20 minutes
Cooking Time: 25 minutes

Ingredients:

- 1 small garlic clove, minced
- ¼ teaspoon dried rosemary, crushed
- ¼ teaspoon dried thyme, crushed
- 1 tablespoon olive oil
- Salt and freshly ground black pepper, to taste
- 1 pound boneless pork shoulder, trimmed and cubed
- 3 tablespoons water
- 2 tablespoons fresh lemon juice

Directions:

1. For pork: in a large bowl, add garlic, dried herbs, oil, salt and black pepper and mix well.
2. Add pork and generously coat with garlic mixture. Keep aside for 15-20 minutes.
3. In the pot of Instant Pot, place pork, water and lemon juice and stir to combine.
4. Secure the lid and cook under "Manual" and "High Pressure" for about 25 minutes.
5. Select the "Cancel" and carefully do a Quick release.
6. Remove the lid and with a slotted spoon, transfer pork into a large bowl.
7. With 2 forks, shred the meat.
8. Top with cooking liquid and serve.

Nutritional Information per Serving:

Calories: 243
Fat: 18.6g
Saturated Fat: 6.3g
Sodium: 80mg
Carbohydrates: 0.4g

Dietary Fiber: 0.1g
Sugar: 0.1g
Protein: 17.7g

Entrée Pork Roast

Makes: 8 servings
Preparation Time: 15 minutes
Cooking Time: 31 minutes

Ingredients:

- 3 garlic cloves, minced
- 1 teaspoon fresh rosemary, minced
- ½ teaspoon chili powder
- Salt and freshly ground black pepper, to taste
- 3-pound pork sirloin tip roast
- 1 tablespoon olive oil
- 1¼ cups water
- 2 tablespoons fresh lemon juice
- 1 tablespoon Erythritol

Directions:

1. In a large bowl, add garlic, rosemary, chili powder, salt and black pepper. Mix well.
2. Add pork and generously coat with garlic mixture.
3. Place the oil in the Instant Pot and select "Sauté". Then add the pork and cook for about 5-6 minutes or until browned completely.

4. Select the "Cancel" and stir in remaining ingredients.
5. Secure the lid and cook under "Manual" and "High Pressure" for about 25 minutes.
6. Select the "Cancel" and carefully do a Natural release for about 10 minutes and then do a Quick release.
7. Remove the lid and transfer roast onto a cutting board.
8. Cut into desires sized slices and serve.

Nutritional Information per Serving:

Calories: 199
Fat: 4.9g
Saturated Fat: 1.8g
Sodium: 368mg
Carbohydrates: 4.1g
Dietary Fiber: 0.2g
Sugar: 3.5g
Protein: 34.8g

Prize Winning Pork Ribs

Makes: 8 servings
Preparation Time: 20 minutes
Cooking Time: 40 minutes

Ingredients:

- 2 garlic cloves, minced
- 1 teaspoon dried thyme, crushed
- 1 teaspoon smoked paprika

- ½ teaspoon ground cumin
- ½ teaspoon ground coriander
- ¼ teaspoon ground allspice
- Salt and freshly ground black pepper, to taste
- 2½ pounds boneless pork ribs
- 1 cup homemade chicken broth
- 1 cup sugar-free tomato sauce
- 2 tablespoons fresh lemon juice
- 2 teaspoons mustard powder
- 2 tablespoons olive oil
- 1 medium yellow onion, sliced

Directions:

1. In a large bowl, mix together garlic, thyme and spices.
2. Add the pork ribs and generously coat with spice mixture.
3. In another small bowl, mix together broth, tomato sauce, lemon juice and mustard.
4. Place the oil in the Instant Pot and select "Sauté". Then add the onion and cook for about 4- 5 minutes.
5. Select "Cancel" and place the ribs over onion and top with broth mixture.
6. Secure the lid and select "Meat" and just use the default time of 35 minutes.
7. Select the "Cancel" and carefully do a Natural release.
8. Remove the lid and serve immediately.

Nutritional Information per Serving:

Calories: 258
Fat: 9.1g
Saturated Fat: 2.3g
Sodium: 358mg
Carbohydrates: 4g
Dietary Fiber: 1.1g

Sugar: 2.2g
Protein: 38.6g

BBQ Party Pork Ribs

Makes: 6 servings
Preparation Time: 15 minutes
Cooking Time: 230 minutes

Ingredients:

- 2 pounds pork baby back ribs
- 2 bay leaves
- 4 garlic cloves, minced
- 2 tablespoons Italian seasoning
- Salt and freshly ground black pepper, to taste
- 4 cups water
- ½ cup sugar-free BBQ sauce

Directions:

1. In the pot of Instant Pot, add all ingredients except BBQ sauce.
2. Secure the lid and cook under "Manual" and "High Pressure" for about 20 minutes.
3. Select the "Cancel" and carefully do a Natural release.
4. Remove the lid and transfer the pork ribs onto a cutting board for about 5 minutes.

5. With paper towels, pat dry the ribs completely.
6. Transfer the ribs into a bowl. Add BBQ sauce and coat the ribs with sauce generously.
7. Cover and refrigerate for about 2-3 hours.
8. Preheat the broiler of oven.
9. Broil the ribs for about 5 minutes per side.
10. Serve immediately.

Nutritional Information per Serving:

Calories: 600
Fat: 46.5g
Saturated Fat: 18.4g
Sodium: 364mg
Carbohydrates: 8.7g
Dietary Fiber: 0.2g
Sugar: 5.9g
Protein: 34.4g

Family Dinner Pork Chops

Makes: 4 servings
Preparation Time: 20 minutes
Cooking Time: 21 minutes

Ingredients:

- 1 tablespoon olive oil
- 2 garlic cloves, minced

- 4 (6-ounce) bone-in pork chops
- Salt and freshly ground black pepper, to taste
- 1 medium onion, chopped
- 1½ cups button mushrooms, chopped roughly
- 1 cup sugar-free tomato sauce
- ½ cup water

Directions:

1. Place the oil in the Instant Pot and select "Sauté". Then add the garlic and cook for about 1 minute.
2. Add pork chops, salt and black pepper and cook for about 5 minutes or until browned from all sides.
3. Select the "Cancel" and stir in remining ingredients.
4. Secure the lid and cook under "Manual" and "High Pressure" for about 15 minutes.
5. Select the "Cancel" and carefully do a Quick release.
6. Remove the lid and serve hot.

Nutritional Information per Serving:

Calories: 608
Fat: 46g
Saturated Fat: 16.4g
Sodium: 483mg
Carbohydrates: 7.3g
Dietary Fiber: 1.8g
Sugar: 4.2g
Protein: 40.3g

Annual Dinner Leg of Lamb

Makes: 10 servings
Preparation Time: 15 minutes
Cooking Time: 1 hour 25 minutes

Ingredients:

- 1 (4-pound) grass-fed bone-in leg of lamb
- Salt and freshly ground black pepper, to taste
- 1 tablespoon olive oil
- 1 large yellow onion, sliced thinly
- 1½ cups homemade chicken broth, divided
- 2 tablespoons fresh lemon juice
- 6 garlic cloves, crushed
- 6 fresh thyme sprigs
- 3 fresh rosemary sprigs

Directions:

1. Generously season the leg of lamb with salt and black pepper.
2. Place the oil in the Instant Pot and select "Sauté". Then add the leg of lamb and sear for about 4 minutes per side or until completely browned.
3. Transfer the lag of lamb into a large plate.
4. Now, add onion and a little salt and cook for about 3 minutes.
5. Add a little broth and cook for about 2 minutes, scraping the brown bits from bottom.
6. Select the "Cancel" and stir in cooked leg of lamb and remaining ingredients.
7. Secure the lid and cook under "Manual" and "High Pressure" for about 75 minutes.
8. Select the "Cancel" and carefully do a Natural release.
9. Remove the lid and with tongs, transfer the leg of lamb onto a cutting board.
10. Cut the leg of lamb into desired slices.

11. Strain the pan liquid into a bowl and pour over sliced leg of lamb, and serve.

Nutritional Information per Serving:
Calories: 365
Fat: 15g
Saturated Fat: 5g
Sodium: 269mg
Carbohydrates: 2.2g
Dietary Fiber: 0.
Sugar: 0.8g
Protein: 52g

Tempting Lamb Shanks

Makes: 2 servings
Preparation Time: 20 minutes
Cooking Time: 23 minutes

Ingredients:

- 2 pounds grass-fed lamb shanks, trimmed
- Salt and freshly ground black pepper, to taste
- 1 tablespoon olive oil
- 10 whole garlic cloves, peeled
- 1 cup homemade chicken broth
- 1 tablespoon sugar-free tomato paste
- ½ teaspoon dried rosemary, crushed
- 2 tablespoons fresh lemon juice
- 1 tablespoon unsalted butter

Directions:

1. Season shanks with salt and pepper.
2. Place the oil in the Instant Pot and select "Sauté". Then add the shanks and sear for about 2-3 minutes per side or until browned completely.
3. Add the garlic cloves and cook for about 1 minute.
4. Select the "Cancel" and stir in remaining ingredients.
5. Secure the lid and cook under "Manual" and "High Pressure" for about 30 minutes.
6. Select the "Cancel" and carefully do a Natural release.
7. Remove the lid and with tongs, transfer the leg of lamb onto a platter.
8. Select "Sauté" and cook for about 5 minutes.
9. Stir in lemon juice and butter until smooth.
10. Pour sauce over shanks and serve.

Nutritional Information per Serving:

Calories: 1007
Fat: 47g
Saturated Fat: 16.9g
Sodium: 858mg
Carbohydrates: 7.5g
Dietary Fiber: 0.9g
Sugar: 1.8g
Protein: 131.3g

Simply Delicious Lamb Chops

Makes: 4 servings
Preparation Time: 15 minutes
Cooking Time: 21 minutes

Ingredients:

- 2 tablespoons butter
- 2 (4-ounce) grass-fed lamb loin chops
- 1 small yellow onion, sliced
- 1 garlic clove, crushed
- 1 (14-ounce) can sugar-free diced tomatoes
- 1 cup homemade chicken broth
- 1½ cups carrots, peeled and sliced
- 1 teaspoon dried rosemary, crushed
- Salt and freshly ground black pepper, to taste
- 2 tablespoons arrowroot starch
- 1 tablespoon cold water

Directions:

1. Place the butter in the Instant Pot and select "Sauté". Then add the chops and sear for about 2-3 minutes per side or until browned completely.
2. Transfer chops onto a platter.
3. Add onion and garlic and cook for about 2-3 minutes.
4. Select the "Cancel" and stir in remaining ingredients.
5. Secure the lid and cook under "Manual" and "High Pressure" for about 10 minutes.
6. Select the "Cancel" and carefully do a Quick release.
7. Meanwhile in a small bowl, dissolve arrowroot starch in cold water.
8. Remove the lid and select the "Sauté".
9. Add arrowroot mixture in Instant Pot, stirring continuously.
10. Cook for about 1-2 minutes.
11. Select the "Cancel" and serve hot.

Nutritional Information per Serving:

Calories: 224
Fat: 10.5g
Saturated Fat: 5.3g
Sodium: 348mg

Carbohydrates: 13.7g
Dietary Fiber: 2.9g
Sugar: 5.6g
Protein: 18.7g

Flavorsome Dinner Meal

Makes: 8 servings
Preparation Time: 15 minutes
Cooking Time: 9 minutes

Ingredients:
- 3 tablespoons butter, divided
- 6 bacon slices, cut into ½-inch pieces
- 1 head cabbage, cored and cut into 1 to 2-inch pieces.
- 2 cups homemade chicken broth
- Salt and freshly ground black pepper, to taste

Directions:
1. Place 1 teaspoon of butter in the Instant Pot and select "Sauté". Then add the bacon and cook for about 4-5 minutes.
2. Add remaining butter and stir until melted completely.
3. Select the "Cancel" and stir in remaining ingredients.
4. Secure the lid and cook under "Manual" and "High Pressure" for about 3 minutes.
5. Select the "Cancel" and carefully do a Quick release
6. Remove the lid and serve hot.

Nutritional Information per Serving:

Calories: 190
Fat: 13.5g
Saturated Fat: 5.8g
Sodium: 747mg
Carbohydrates: 7.1g
Dietary Fiber: 2.8g
Sugar: 3.8g
Protein: 2.5

Bacon with Veggies

Makes: 6 servings
Preparation Time: 20 minutes
Cooking Time: 14 minutes

Ingredients:

- 1 pound fresh green beans, trimmed
- ½ teaspoon butter
- 6 ounces bacon, chopped
- ½ of yellow onion, chopped
- 8 ounces fresh mushrooms, sliced
- 1 garlic clove, minced
- 1 teaspoon fresh lemon juice
- Salt and freshly ground black pepper, to taste

Directions:

1. In the pot of Instant Pot, place green beans and enough water to barely cover the beans.

2. Secure the lid and cook under "Manual" and "High Pressure" for about 1-2 minutes.
3. Select the "Cancel" and carefully do a Quick release
4. Drain green beans into a colander and set aside.
5. Place butter in the Instant Pot and select "Sauté". Then add the bacon and cook for about 4-5 minutes.
6. Add onions and garlic and cook for about 1 minute.
7. Add mushrooms and cook for about 4-5 minutes.
8. Stir in green beans, lemon juice, salt and black pepper and cook for about 1-2 minutes.
9. Select the "Cancel" and serve hot.

Nutritional Information per Serving:

Calories: 192
Fat: 12.4g
Saturated Fat: 4.1g
Sodium: 692mg
Carbohydrates: 8.1g
Dietary Fiber: 3.2g
Sugar: 2.1g
Protein: 3.2g

Instant Pot Seafood Recipes

Super-Quick Salmon

Makes: 6 servings
Preparation Time: 10 minutes
Cooking Time: 3 minutes

Ingredients:

- 2 (5-ounce) salmon fillets
- 2 teaspoons fresh lemon juice
- 2 lemon slices
- Salt and freshly ground black pepper, to taste

Directions:

1. Arrange the trivet in the bottom of Instant Pot. Add 1½ cups of water in Instant Pot.
2. Season salmon fillets with salt and black pepper and drizzle with lemon juice evenly.
3. Place the salmon fillets on top of trivet in a single layer. Arrange 1 lemon slice over each fillet.
4. Secure the lid and select "Steam" and just use the default time of 3 minutes.
5. Select the "Cancel" and carefully do a Quick release.
6. Remove the lid and serve hot.

Nutritional Information per Serving:

Calories: 63
Fat: 2.9g
Saturated Fat: 0.4g

Sodium: 48mg
Carbohydrates: 0.2g
Dietary Fiber: 0.1g
Sugar: 0.1g
Protein: 9.2g

Deliciously Tangy Salmon

Makes: 4 servings
Preparation Time: 20 minutes
Cooking Time: 7 minutes

Ingredients:

- 4 (4-ounce) salmon fillets
- 1 teaspoon garlic, minced
- 1 teaspoon fresh lemon zest, grated finely
- 1 cup homemade chicken broth
- 1 tablespoon olive oil
- 2 tablespoons fresh lemon juice
- Salt and freshly ground black pepper, to taste

Directions:

1. In the pot of Instant Pot, add all ingredients and mix.
2. Secure the lid and cook under "Manual" and "High Pressure" for about 7 minutes.
3. Select the "Cancel" and carefully do a Natural release.
4. Remove the lid and serve the salmon fillets with the topping of cooking sauce.

Nutritional Information per Serving:
Calories: 192
Fat: 10.9g
Saturated Fat: 1.7g
Sodium: 281mg
Carbohydrates: 0.7g
Dietary Fiber: 0.1g
Sugar: 0.4g
Protein: 23.3g

Nutritious Salmon Dinner

Makes: 4 servings
Preparation Time: 10 minutes
Cooking Time: 2 minutes

Ingredients:

- 1 garlic clove, minced
- 1 teaspoon powdered stevia
- 1 tablespoon red chili powder
- 1 teaspoon ground cumin
- Salt and freshly ground black pepper, to taste
- 1 pound salmon fillet, cut into 4 pieces.

Directions:

1. Arrange the trivet in the bottom of Instant Pot. Add 1½ cups of water in Instant Pot.
2. In a small bowl, mix together all ingredients except salmon.
3. Rub salmon pieces with spice mixture evenly.
4. Place the salmon fillets on top of trivet in a single layer. Arrange 1 lemon slice over each fillet.
5. Secure the lid and select "Steam" and just use the default time of 2 minutes.
6. Select the "Cancel" and carefully do a Quick release.
7. Remove the lid and serve hot.

Nutritional Information per Serving:

Calories: 159
Fat: 7.4g
Saturated Fat: 1.1g
Sodium: 109mg
Carbohydrates: 1.5g
Dietary Fiber: 0.7g
Sugar: 0.2g
Protein: 22.4g

Wholesome Salmon Meal

Makes: 4 servings
Preparation Time: 15 minutes
Cooking Time: 3 minutes

Ingredients:

- ¼ cup olive oil
- 2 tablespoons fresh lemon juice

- 1 garlic clove, minced
- 1 tablespoon feta cheese, crumbled
- ¼ teaspoon dried oregano
- Salt and freshly ground black pepper, to taste
- 1 pound salmon fillets
- 2 fresh rosemary sprigs
- 2 lemon slices

Directions:

1. In a large bowl, add oil, lemon juice, garlic, feta, oregano, salt and black pepper and beat until well co combined.
2. Arrange the trivet in the bottom of Instant Pot. Add 1½ cups of water in Instant Pot.
3. Place the salmon fillets on top of trivet in a single layer and top with dressing. Arrange1 rosemary sprig and 1 lemon slice over each fillet.
4. Secure the lid and select "Steam" and just use the default time of 3 minutes.
5. Select the "Cancel" and carefully do a Quick release.
6. Remove the lid and serve hot.

Nutritional Information per Serving:

Calories: 270
Fat: 20.3g
Saturated Fat: 3.3g
Sodium: 117mg
Carbohydrates: 1.1g
Dietary Fiber: 0.4g
Sugar: 0.3g
Protein: 22.5g

Healthier Mahi-Mahi

Makes: 2 servings
Preparation Time: 15 minutes
Cooking Time: 7 minutes

Ingredients:

- 2 (4-ounce) mahi-mahi fillets
- Salt and freshly ground black pepper, to taste
- 2 garlic cloves, minced
- 2 tablespoons fresh lime juice
- 2 tablespoons erythritol
- 1 teaspoon red pepper flakes, crushed

Directions:

1. Season mahi-mahi with salt and black pepper evenly.
2. In a bowl, mix together remaining ingredients.
3. Arrange the trivet in the bottom of Instant Pot. Add 1 cup of water in Instant Pot.
4. Place the fish fillets on top of trivet in a single layer and top with sauce.
5. Secure the lid and select "Steam" and just use the default time of 5 minutes.
6. Select the "Cancel" and carefully do a Quick release.
7. Remove the lid and serve hot.

Nutritional Information per Serving:
Calories: 109
Fat: 1.2g
Saturated Fat: 0g
Sodium: 189mg
Carbohydrates: 17.6g
Dietary Fiber: 0.3g

Sugar: 15.1g
Protein: 21.4g

Lively Flavored Mahi-Mahi

Makes: 6 servings
Preparation Time: 15 minutes
Cooking Time: 14 minutes

Ingredients:

- 3 tablespoons butter
- 1 (28-ounce) can sugar-free diced tomatoes
- 1 yellow onion, sliced
- 2 tablespoons fresh lemon juice
- 1 teaspoon dried oregano
- Salt and freshly ground black pepper, to taste
- 6 (4-ounce) mahi-mahi fillets

Directions:

1. Place the butter in the Instant Pot and select "Sauté". Then add all ingredients except fish fillets and cook for about 8-
2. 10 minutes.
3. Select the "Cancel" and place fish fillets over sauce. With a spoon, place some sauce over fillets.
4. Secure the lid and cook under "Manual" and "High Pressure" for about 4 minutes.
5. Select the "Cancel" and carefully do a Quick release.
6. Remove the lid and serve hot with the topping of sauce.

Nutritional Information per Serving:

Calories: 184
Fat: 7.1g
Saturated Fat: 3.7g
Sodium: 187mg
Carbohydrates: 8.2g
Dietary Fiber: 2.1g
Sugar: 4.4g
Protein: 22.6g

Foolproof Cod Parcel

Makes: 6 servings
Preparation Time: 15 minutes
Cooking Time: 5 minutes

Ingredients:

- 2 (4-ounce) cod fillets
- ½ teaspoon garlic powder
- Salt and freshly ground black pepper, to taste
- 2 fresh dill sprigs
- 4 lemon slices
- 2 tablespoons butter

Directions:

1. Arrange 2 large parchment squares onto a smooth surface.
2. Place 1 fillet in the center of each parchment square and sprinkle with garlic powder, salt and black pepper.
3. Top each fillet with 1 dill sprig, 2 lemon slices and 1 tablespoon of butter.

4. Fold each parchment paper around the fillets to seal.
5. Arrange the trivet in the bottom of Instant Pot. Add 1 cup of water in Instant Pot.
6. Place the fish parcels on top of trivet in a single layer.
7. Secure the lid and cook under "Manual" and "High Pressure" for about 5 minutes.
8. Select the "Cancel" and carefully do a Quick release.
9. Remove the lid and transfer fish parcels onto serving plates.
10. Unwrap the parcels and serve.

Nutritional Information per Serving:

Calories: 196
Fat: 12.6g
Saturated Fat: 7.3g
Sodium: 230mg
Carbohydrates: 0.8g
Dietary Fiber: 0.2g
Sugar: 0.3g
Protein: 20.5g

Energizing Cod Platter

Makes: 4 servings
Preparation Time: 20 minutes
Cooking Time: 5 minutes

Ingredients:

- 1 pound cherry tomatoes, halved
- 2 tablespoons fresh rosemary, chopped

- 4 (4-ounce) cod fillets
- 2 garlic cloves, minced
- 1 tablespoon olive oil
- Salt and freshly ground black pepper, to taste

Directions:

1. Place half of cherry tomatoes in the bottom of a large, greased heatproof bowl, followed by the rosemary.
2. Arrange cod fillets on top in a single layer, followed by the remaining tomatoes.
3. Sprinkle with garlic and drizzle with oil.
4. Arrange the bowl into Instant Pot.
5. Secure the lid and cook under "Manual" and "High Pressure" for about 5 minutes.
6. Select the "Cancel" and carefully do a Quick release.
7. Remove the lid and transfer the fish fillets and tomatoes in serving plates.
8. Sprinkle with salt and black pepper and serve.

Nutritional Information per Serving:

Calories: 149
Fat: 5g
Saturated Fat: 0.7g
Sodium: 116mg
Carbohydrates: 6g
Dietary Fiber: 2.1g
Sugar: 3g
Protein: 21.4g

Luscious Cod Meal

Makes: 6 servings
Preparation Time: 20 minutes
Cooking Time: 22 minutes

Ingredients:

- 2 tablespoons coconut oil
- 1 mediumonion, chopped finely
- 1 garlic clove, minced
- 2 large carrots, peeled and chopped
- 2 cupscanned sugar-free chopped tomatoes with juice
- 2 tablespoonsfresh parsley, chopped
- 2 cups water
- 1 lb. frozen cod fillets
- Salt and freshly ground black pepper, to taste
- 2½ cupsfresh kale, trimmed and chopped
- ½ cupheavy cream

Directions:

1. Place the coconut oil in the Instant Pot and select "Sauté". Then add the onion and garlic and cook for about 3 minutes.
2. Add carrots, tomatoes, parsley and water and cook for about 3-4 minutes.
3. Select the "Cancel" and arrange a steamer basket on top.
4. Place cod fillets into steamer basket and sprinkle with salt and black pepper.
5. Secure the lid and cook under "Manual" and "High Pressure" for about 6 minutes.
6. Select the "Cancel" and carefully do a Quick release.
7. Remove the lid and carefully, transfer the fish fillets onto a platter.
8. With an immersion blender, puree the carrot mixture.
9. Select "Sauté" and stir in kale and cream and cook for about 5 minutes.

10. Stir in fish fillets and cook for about 3-4 minutes.

Nutritional Information per Serving:

Calories: 177
Fat: 9.1g
Saturated Fat: 6.2g
Sodium: 111mg
Carbohydrates: 9.9g
Dietary Fiber: 2.2g
Sugar: 3.6g
Protein: 15.5g

Elegant Dinner Mussels

Makes: 4 servings
Preparation Time: 20 minutes
Cooking Time: 7 minutes

Ingredients:

- 1 tablespoon olive oil
- 1 medium yellow onion, chopped
- 1 garlic clove, minced
- ½ teaspoon dried rosemary, crushed
- 1 cup homemade chicken broth
- 2 tablespoons fresh lemon juice
- Salt and freshly ground black pepper, to taste
- 2 pounds mussels, cleaned and de-bearded

Directions:

1. Place the oil in the Instant Pot and select "Sauté". Then add the onion and cook for about 5 minutes.
2. Add garlic and rosemary and cook for about 1 minute.
3. Select "Cancel" and stir in the broth, lemon juice and black pepper.
4. Place the mussels in steamer trivet and arrange the trivet in Instant Pot.
5. Secure the lid and cook under "Manual" and "Low Pressure" for about 1 minute.
6. Select the "Cancel" and carefully do a Quick release.
7. Remove the lid and transfer the mussels into serving bowl.
8. Top with the cooking liquid and serve.

Nutritional Information per Serving:

Calories: 249
Fat: 9g
Saturated Fat: 1.6g
Sodium: 881mg
Carbohydrates: 11.7g
Dietary Fiber: 0.7g
Sugar: 1.5g
Protein: 28.6g

3-Ingredients Lobster Dinner

Makes: 2 servings
Preparation Time: 20 minutes
Cooking Time: 3 minutes

Ingredients:

- 2 pound lobster tails, cut in half
- 2 tablespoons unsalted butter, melted
- Pinch of salt

Directions:

1. Arrange the steamer trivet in the bottom of Instant Pot. Add 1 cup of water in Instant Pot.
2. Arrange the lobster tails, shell side in trivet.
3. Secure the lid and cook under "Manual" and "Low Pressure" for about 3 minutes.
4. Select the "Cancel" and carefully do a Quick release.
5. Remove the lid and transfer the tails in serving plate.
6. Drizzle with butter and sprinkle with salt before serving.

Nutritional Information per Serving:

Calories: 507
Fat: 15.3g
Saturated Fat: 8.2g
Sodium: 2000mg
Carbohydrates: 0g
Dietary Fiber: 0g
Sugar: 0g
Protein: 86.3g

Deliciously Creamy Lobster

Makes: 2 servings
Preparation Time: 20 minutes
Cooking Time: 3 minutes

Ingredients:

- 1½ cups water
- 1 teaspoon old bay seasoning
- 2 pound fresh lobster tails
- 1 scallion, chopped
- ½ cup mayonnaise
- 2 tablespoons unsalted butter, melted
- 2 tablespoons fresh lemon juice, divided

Directions:

1. Arrange the steamer trivet in the bottom of Instant Pot. Add water and 1-2 pinches of old bay seasoning in Instant Pot.
2. Arrange lobster tail on top of trivet, shell side down, meat side up.
3. Drizzle lobster tails with 1 tablespoon of lemon juice.
4. Secure the lid and cook under "Manual" and "High Pressure" for about 3 minutes.
5. Select the "Cancel" and carefully do a Quick release.
6. Remove the lid and transfer the tails into the bowl of ice bath.
7. Lay in for a minute.
8. With kitchen shears, cut the underbelly of the tail down the center.
9. Remove the meat and chop it up into large chunks.
10. In a large bowl, add lobster meat, scallions, mayonnaise, butter, seasoning and lemon juice and mix well.
11. Refrigerate for at least 15 minutes before serving.

Nutritional Information per Serving:

Calories: 740
Fat: 35g
Saturated Fat: 11.2g
Sodium: 3000mg
Carbohydrates: 14.4g
Dietary Fiber: 0.1g
Sugar: 4.1g
Protein: 87g

Special Occasion's Crab Legs

Makes: 3 servings
Preparation Time: 20 minutes
Cooking Time: 4 minutes

Ingredients:

- 1½ pounds frozen crab legs
- Salt, to taste
- 2 tablespoons butter, melted

Directions:

1. Arrange the trivet in the bottom of Instant Pot. Add 1 cup of water and about teaspoon of salt in Instant Pot.
2. Place the crab legs on top of trivet and sprinkle with salt.
3. Secure the lid and cook under "Manual" and "High Pressure" for about 4 minutes.

4. Select the "Cancel" and carefully do a Quick release.
5. Remove the lid and transfer crab legs onto a serving platter.
6. Drizzle with butter and serve.

Nutritional Information per Serving:

Calories: 297
Fat: 11.1g
Saturated Fat: 4.9g
Sodium: 2500mg
Carbohydrates: 0g
Dietary Fiber: 0g
Sugar: 0g
Protein: 43.6g

Instant Pot Veggie Recipes

Versatile Cauliflower Dish

Makes: 5 servings
Preparation Time: 20 minutes
Cooking Time: 14 minutes

Ingredients:

For Sauce:

- 6-ounces goat cheese
- 1/3 cup heavy cream
- 1 tablespoon olive oil
- 1 teaspoon ground nutmeg
- Salt and ground white pepper, to taste

For Cauliflower:

- 1 (2 pound) head cauliflower
- 1 cup homemade vegetable broth
- 2 tablespoons fresh lemon juice
- 2 tablespoons olive oil
- 2 teaspoons red pepper flakes, crushed
- Salt to taste

Directions:

1. For sauce: in a food processor, add all ingredients and pulse until smooth. Set aside until serving.
2. In the pot of Instant Pot, place cauliflower head and top with remaining ingredients.

3. Secure the lid and cook under "Manual" and "High Pressure" for about 10 minutes.
4. Select the "Cancel" and carefully do a Quick release.
5. Preheat the broiler of oven.
6. Remove the lid and transfer the cauliflower head onto a cutting board.
7. Cut cauliflower head into pieces and place onto a broiler pan.
8. Broil for about 3-4 minutes or until golden brown.
9. Remove from oven and serve with the topping of cheese sauce.

Nutritional Information per Serving:

Calories: 312
Fat: 24.3g
Saturated Fat: 11.7g
Sodium: 360mg
Carbohydrates: 11.5g
Dietary Fiber: 4.9g
Sugar: 5.6g
Protein: 15.3g

Easy-to-Prepare Broccoli

Makes: 4 servings
Preparation Time: 15 minutes
Cooking Time: 5 minutes

Ingredients:

- 1 pound broccoli florets
- 2 tablespoons butter, melted

- Salt and freshly ground black pepper, to taste

Directions:

1. Arrange the trivet in the bottom of Instant Pot. Add 1 cup of water in Instant Pot.
2. Place the broccoli florets on top of trivet in a single layer.
3. Secure the lid and cook under "Manual" and "High Pressure" for 3-5 minutes.
4. Select the "Cancel" and carefully do a Quick release.
5. Remove the lid and transfer broccoli onto a serving platter.
6. Drizzle with butter and sprinkle with salt and black pepper.
7. Serve immediately.

Nutritional Information per Serving:

Calories: 90
Fat: 6.1g
Saturated Fat: 3.7g
Sodium: 117mg
Carbohydrates: 7.6g
Dietary Fiber: 3g
Sugar: 1.9g
Protein: 3.2g

Nutty Brussels Sprouts

Makes: 4 servings
Preparation Time: 15 minutes
Cooking Time: 3 minutes

Ingredients:

- 1 pound Brussels sprouts, trimmed and halved
- ½ tablespoon unsalted butter, melted
- ½ cup almonds, chopped

Directions:

1. Arrange the steamer trivet in the bottom of Instant Pot. Add 1 cup of water to the Instant Pot.
2. Arrange the Brussels sprout on top of trivet.
3. Secure the lid and cook under "Manual" and "High Pressure" for about 3 minutes.
4. Select the "Cancel" and carefully do a Quick release.
5. Remove the lid and transfer the Brussels sprouts onto serving plates.
6. Drizzle with the melted butter.
7. Top with almonds and serve.

Nutritional Information per Serving:

Calories: 130
Fat: 7.8g
Saturated Fat: 1.5g
Sodium: 39mg
Carbohydrates: 12.9g
Dietary Fiber: 5.7g
Sugar: 3g
Protein: 6.4g

Refreshing Luncheon Green Beans

Makes: 4 servings
Preparation Time: 10 minutes
Cooking Time: 5 minutes

Ingredients:

- 1poundfresh green beans
- 2tablespoonsbutter
- 1garlic clove, minced
- Salt and freshly ground black pepper, to taste
- 1½ cups water

Directions:

1. In the pot of Instant Pot, add all ingredients and stir to combine.
2. Secure the lid and cook under "Manual" and "Low Pressure" for about 5 minutes.
3. Select the "Cancel" and carefully do a Quick release.
4. Remove the lid and serve hot.

Nutritional Information per Serving:

Calories: 87
Fat: 5.9g
Saturated Fat: 3.7g
Sodium: 96mg
Carbohydrates: 8.4g
Dietary Fiber: 3.9g
Sugar: 1.6g
Protein: 2.2g

Nutritive Spinach Plate

Makes: 6 servings
Preparation Time: 15 minutes
Cooking Time: 12 minutes

Ingredients:

- 2 tablespoons olive oil
- 1 medium yellow onion, chopped
- 1 tablespoon garlic, minced
- 10 cups fresh spinach, chopped
- 1 cup tomatoes, chopped
- ½ cup sugar-free tomato puree
- 1¼ cups homemade vegetable broth
- 1 tablespoon fresh lemon juice
- ½ teaspoon red pepper flakes, crushed
- Salt and freshly ground black pepper, to taste

Directions:

1. Place the oil in the Instant Pot and select "Sauté". Then add the onion and cook for about 3 minutes.
2. Add garlic and red pepper flakes and cook for about 1 minute.
3. Add spinach and cook for about 2 minutes.
4. Select "Cancel" and stir in the remaining ingredients.
5. Next, secure the lid and cook under "Manual" and "High Pressure" for about 6 minutes.
6. Select the "Cancel" and carefully do a Quick release.
7. Remove the lid and serve warm.

Nutritional Information per Serving:

Calories: 83
Fat: 5.3g
Saturated Fat: 0.8g
Sodium: 207mg
Carbohydrates: 7.4g
Dietary Fiber: 2.3g
Sugar: 3g
Protein: 3.4g

Yummiest Glazed Carrot

Makes: 4 servings
Preparation Time: 20 minutes
Cooking Time: 3 minutes

Ingredients:

- 1 pound carrots
- 2 tablespoons butter
- 2 tablespoons Erythritol
- 2 tablespoons Dijon mustard
- 2 teaspoons garlic, minced
- 1 teaspoon ground cumin
- 1 teaspoon paprika
- Salt and freshly ground black pepper, to taste
- Dash of hot sauce

Directions:

1. Cut the carrots into quarters lengthwise and then cut each quarter in half.
2. Arrange the steamer trivet in the bottom of Instant Pot. Add 1 cup of the water in Instant Pot.
3. Arrange the carrots on top of trivet.
4. Secure the lid and cook under "Manual" and "High Pressure" for about 1 minute.
5. Select the "Cancel" and carefully do a Quick release.
6. Remove the lid and transfer carrots onto a plate.
7. Remove water from Instant Pot.
8. Place the butter in the Instant Pot and select "Sauté". Then add the remaining ingredients and stir to combine.
9. Select the "Cancel" and stir in the carrots.
10. Serve warm.

Nutritional Information per Serving:

Calories: 108
Fat: 6.3g
Saturated Fat: 3.7g
Sodium: 252mg
Carbohydrates: 20.1g
Dietary Fiber: 3.4g
Sugar: 13.2g
Protein: 1.6g

Super-Food Veggie Platter

Makes: 6 servings
Preparation Time: 20 minutes
Cooking Time: 14 minutes

Ingredients:

- 1 tablespoon olive oil
- ½ small yellow onion, chopped
- 3 medium carrots, peeled and cut into ½-inch slices
- 4 garlic cloves, minced
- 10-ounces fresh kale, trimmed and chopped
- ½ cup homemade vegetable broth
- Salt and freshly ground black pepper, to taste
- 1 tablespoon fresh lemon juice
- Pinch of red pepper flakes, crushed

Directions:

1. Place the oil in the Instant Pot and select "Sauté". Then add the onion and carrot and cook for about 5 minutes.
2. Add garlic and cook for about 1 minute.
3. Select the "Cancel" and stir in kale, broth, salt and black pepper.
4. Secure the lid and cook under "Manual" and "High Pressure" for about 8 minutes.
5. Select the "Cancel" and carefully do a Quick release.
6. Remove the lid and stir in lemon juice.
7. Transfer the vegetable mixture into serving plate.
8. Serve with the sprinkling of red pepper flakes.

Nutritional Information per Serving:

Calories: 65
Fat: 2.5g
Saturated Fat: 0.4g
Sodium: 133mg
Carbohydrates: 9.3g
Dietary Fiber: 1.7g
Sugar: 1.9g
Protein: 2.3g

Beautiful Colored Veggies

Makes: 8 servings
Preparation Time: 20 minutes
Cooking Time: 7 minutes

Ingredients:

- 1 tablespoon olive oil
- 2 small yellow onions, chopped roughly
- 2 garlic cloves, minced
- 6 medium zucchinis, chopped roughly
- 1 lb. cherry tomatoes
- 1 cup water
- Salt and freshly ground black pepper, to taste
- 2 tablespoons fresh basil, chopped

Directions:

1. Place the oil in the Instant Pot and select "Sauté". Then add the onion and garlic and cook for about 3-4 minutes.
2. Add zucchinis and tomatoes and cook for about 1-2 minutes.
3. Select the "Cancel" and stir in remaining ingredients except basil.
4. Secure the lid and cook under "Manual" and "High Pressure" for about 5 minutes.
5. Select the "Cancel" and carefully do a Natural release.
6. Remove the lid and transfer the vegetable mixture onto a serving platter.
7. Garnish with basil and serve.

Nutritional Information per Serving:

Calories: 76
Fat: 2.9g

Saturated Fat: 0.4g
Sodium: 53mg
Carbohydrates: 12.1g
Dietary Fiber: 3.6g
Sugar: 6.4g
Protein: 3.4g

Flavorful Veggies Dish

Makes: 8 servings
Preparation Time: 20 minutes
Cooking Time: 8 minutes

Ingredients:

- 1 tablespoon olive oil
- 12-ounces fresh mushrooms, sliced
- 1 cup onion, chopped
- 2 garlic cloves, minced
- 4 medium zucchinis, cut into ½-inch slices
- 2 tablespoons fresh basil, chopped
- Salt and freshly ground black pepper, to taste
- 1 (15-ounce) can sugar-free crushed tomatoes with juice

Directions:

1. Place the oil in the Instant Pot and select "Sauté". Then add the mushrooms, onion and garlic and cook for about 5 minutes.

2. Add the zucchinis, basil, salt and black pepper and cook for about 1-2 minutes.
3. Select the "Cancel" and place tomatoes with juice on top of vegetable mixture.
4. Secure the lid and cook under "Manual" and "Low Pressure" for about 1 minute.
5. Select the "Cancel" and carefully do a Natural release.
6. Remove the lid and serve hot.

Nutritional Information per Serving:

Calories: 68
Fat: 2.1g
Saturated Fat: 0.3g
Sodium: 134mg
Carbohydrates: 10.6g
Dietary Fiber: 3.6g
Sugar: 6g
Protein: 4g

Meatless Dinner Casserole

Makes: 8 servings
Preparation Time: 20 minutes
Cooking Time: 30 minutes

Ingredients:

- ½ cup unsweetened almond milk

- ½ cup almond flour
- 8 large organic eggs
- Salt and freshly ground black pepper, to taste
- 1 cup tomato, chopped
- 1 medium zucchini, chopped
- 1 medium green bell pepper, seeded and chopped
- 1½ cups mozzarella cheese, shredded

Directions:

1. Arrange the trivet in the bottom of Instant Pot. Add 1 cup of water in Instant Pot.
2. In a heatproof bowl, add milk, flour, eggs, salt and black pepper and beat until well combined.
3. Add vegetables and 1 cup of cheese and stir to combine.
4. With a piece of foil, cover the bowl and place on top of trivet.
5. Secure the lid and cook under "Manual" and "High Pressure" for about 30 minutes.
6. Select the "Cancel" and carefully do a Natural release for about 10 minutes and then do a Quick release.
7. Remove the lid and serve immediately.

Nutritional Information per Serving:

Calories: 102
Fat: 9.6g
Saturated Fat: 2.4g
Sodium: 139mg
Carbohydrates: 5.1g
Dietary Fiber: 1.6g
Sugar: 2.2g
Protein: 10g

Cauliflower Rice

Makes: 4 servings
Preparation Time: 20 minutes
Cooking Time: 14 minutes

Ingredients:

- 1 medium head cauliflower, chop into large pieces
- 2 tablespoons olive oil
- ½ teaspoon dried parsley
- ¼ teaspoon ground cumin
- ¼ teaspoon paprika
- ¼ teaspoon ground turmeric
- Salt, to taste
- 2 tablespoons fresh parsley, chopped

Directions:

1. Arrange the trivet in the bottom of Instant Pot. Add 1 cup of water in Instant Pot.
2. Place cauliflower pieces on top of trivet.
3. Secure the lid and cook under "Manual" and "High Pressure" for about 10 minutes.
4. Select the "Cancel" and carefully do a Quick release.
5. Remove the lid and transfer the cauliflower onto a plate.
6. Remove water from Instant Pot.
7. Place the oil in the Instant Pot and select "Sauté". Then add the cooked cauliflower and with a spoon, break into smaller chunks.
8. Add spices and cook for about 1-2 minutes.
9. Select the "Cancel" and serve hot.

Nutritional Information per Serving:

Calories: 118
Fat: 7.3g
Saturated Fat: 1g
Sodium: 107mg
Carbohydrates: 12.3g
Dietary Fiber: 5.8g
Sugar: 5.5g
Protein: 4.5g

Cauliflower Mash

Makes: 6 servings
Preparation Time: 20 minutes
Cooking Time: 14 minutes

Ingredients:

- 1 large head cauliflower, chop into large pieces
- 1 tablespoon butter, softened
- 1 garlic clove, minced
- 2 teaspoons fresh chives, minced
- Salt and freshly ground black pepper, to taste

Directions:

1. Arrange the trivet in the bottom of Instant Pot. Add 1 cup of water in Instant Pot.
2. Place cauliflower pieces on top of trivet.

3. Secure the lid and cook under "Manual" and "High Pressure" for about 5 minutes.
4. Select the "Cancel" and carefully do a Quick release.
5. Remove the lid and transfer the cauliflower pieces into a bowl.
6. Add remaining ingredients and with an immersion hand blender, blend until desired texture is achieved.
7. Serve immediately.

Nutritional Information per Serving:

Calories: 65
Fat: 2.1g
Saturated Fat: 1.3g
Sodium: 98mg
Carbohydrates: 10.2g
Dietary Fiber: 8.4g
Sugar: 4.5g
Protein: 3.8g

Carrot Mash

Makes: 4 servings
Preparation Time: 20 minutes
Cooking Time: 4 minutes

Ingredients:
- 1½ pound carrots, peeled and chopped roughly
- 1 tablespoon butter, softened
- 1 teaspoon Erythritol

- Salt, to taste

Directions:

1. Arrange the trivet in the bottom of Instant Pot. Add 1 cup of water in Instant Pot.
2. Place carrot pieces on top of trivet.
3. Secure the lid and cook under "Manual" and "High Pressure" for about 4 minutes.
4. Select the "Cancel" and carefully do a Quick release.
5. Remove the lid and transfer the carrots into a bowl.
6. Add remaining ingredients and with an immersion hand blender, blend until desired texture is achieved.
7. Serve immediately.

Nutritional Information per Serving:

Calories: 95
Fat: 2.9g
Saturated Fat: 1.8g
Sodium: 176mg
Carbohydrates: 18g
Dietary Fiber: 4.2g
Sugar: 9.6g
Protein: 1.4g

CPSIA information can be obtained
at www.ICGtesting.com
Printed in the USA
BVOW04s1149040118

504467BV00003B/13/P

9 781981 458301